Rehabilitation Institute *of* Chicago

THE
Back
Pain
BOOK

 REVISED 2ND EDITION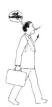

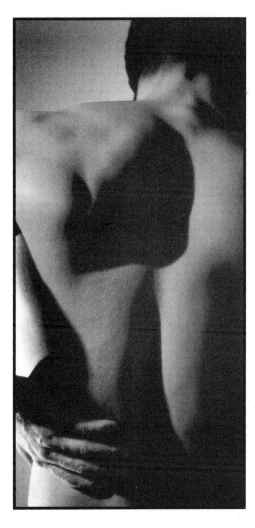

D1390646

THE BACK PAIN BOOK was developed through the Rehabilitation Institute of Chicago (RIC) and is currently used for patient education by its Pain Program. Ranked the "Best Rehabilitation Hospital in America" by *U.S. News & World Report* every year since 1991, RIC strives to help people of all ages achieve the best life possible through excellence in patient care, rehabilitation research, advanced professional education, advocacy for people with disabilities, and community service. Through its network of over thirty locations in Chicago and the Midwest, RIC provides inpatient, day rehabilitation, and outpatient care on many levels—from brain and spinal cord injuries and stroke to arthritis, chronic pain, and sports injuries. RIC's services go beyond the traditional bounds of medical care to address every aspect of rehabilitation—helping people regain everyday life skills, return to work or school, or participate in sports and fitness programs that promote physical well-being—giving patients their best hope of returning to fulfilling lives.

Rehabilitation Institute *of* Chicago

THE
Back
Pain
BOOK

 REVISED 2ND EDITION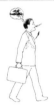

A SELF-HELP GUIDE FOR DAILY RELIEF OF NECK AND LOW BACK PAIN

Mike Hage

Revised by Jo Fasen, Sharon Feldmann, Bill Keeley,
Annie O'Connor, Virginia Wirth-Pattullo

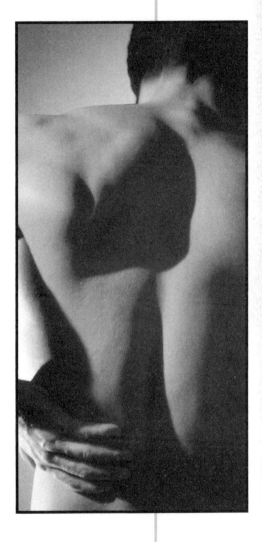

Ω
PEACHTREE
ATLANTA

*To my parents George and Nellie, to J. D. Meacham, M. K., De-de,
and George: you taught me that painful things are not the enemy, but the
signal—announcing that it's time to change, to improve, to heal, and to
embrace your life.*

—MIKE HAGE (original dedication)

*To the memory of Mike Hage: Mike taught us that compassion,
communication and a willingness to share ideas and experiences are the
essential qualities a physical therapist needs to assist people in overcoming
pain and functional loss. Having experienced the impact the first edition of
THE BACK PAIN BOOK had on our patients, it is our pleasure to share our
knowledge and ideas by contributing to this valuable resource.*

—THE REVISION AUTHORS

Published by
PEACHTREE PUBLISHERS
1700 Chattahoochee Avenue
Atlanta, GA 30318-2112

www.peachtree-online.com

Text © 1992, 2005 Rehabilitation Institute of Chicago
Illustrations © 1992 Rehabilitation Institute of Chicago; © 2005 Karen Dirr

Medical illustrations by Karen Dirr, MAMS
Book design by Regina Dalton-Fischel
Composition by Robin Sherman

Production Editor: Elizabeth W. Snow

Manufactured in the United States of America
10 9 8 7 6 5 4 3 2 1

Library of Congress Cataloging-in-Publication Data

The back pain book : a self-help guide for daily relief of neck and low back pain / written by Mike Hage
... [et al.] ; illustrated by Karen Dirr.-- 2nd ed.
    p. cm.
Rev. ed. of: Back pain book / Mike Hage. c1992.
Includes bibliographical references.
ISBN 1-56145-342-0
1. Backache--Popular works. 2. Neck pain--Popular works. I. Hage, Mike, 1954- II. Hage, Mike, 1954-
Back pain book. III. Title.

RD771.B217B318 2004
617.5'64--dc22

2004027732

CONTENTS

CHAPTER 3
GOOD MOVES/BAD MOVES DURING DAILY ACTIVITIES

CHAPTER 4
WHEEL OF FUNCTION

CHAPTER 5
STRATEGIC EXERCISES

FOREWORD

Great ideas, innovations and works of writing stand the test of time. Mike Hage's BACK PAIN BOOK is one of these works. It has taken the very complex and multifactorial problem of low back pain, explained it, and provided the reader with information and knowledge to address the problem. Low back pain or neck pain will affect almost all of us at some point in our lives. Most of us get better with very little to no intervention. Many, however, do not. The staggering cost of low back care continues to rise each decade. Misinformation, fear, and avoidance are major obstacles to improving symptoms. The remedies provided in THE BACK PAIN BOOK are clear and the explanations and directions, accurate and concise.

Mike Hage was an exceptional person and physical therapist. He saw beauty in the movement of the human body and studied to learn all he could about that movement. In working with back and neck patients, Mike learned that certain movement patterns could help reduce their symptoms. In his first edition of THE BACK PAIN BOOK, he integrated this knowledge into five easy-to-read and easy-to-understand chapters designed to help average back pain sufferers take control of their problem by providing the knowledge they need to overcome the symptoms and prevent reccurrences of low back and neck pain. He taught us, in simple terms, how to be smarter with respect to our backs.

Mike Hage passed away in 2000. His passion for patient care, his knowledge, and his understanding of people in general and spinal care in particular have greatly influenced his colleagues. Five of those colleagues—Bill Keeley, Annie O'Connor, Virginia Wirth-Pattullo, Sharon Feldmann, and Jo Fasen—

joined together to honor Mike's career and his dedication to patients with low back and neck pain by taking a truly remarkable book and updating it to reflect an even more functional approach to low back pain care.

With this second edition of THE BACK PAIN BOOK, Mike Hage's legacy of caring and compassion for patients with low back and neck pain, along with the ideas and approaches of some of the best physical therapists from the best rehabilitation hospital in the country, is further solidified. All patients with low back pain can read this book and get clear, concise, and practical information that can help them alleviate and prevent low back pain in their daily lives.

JOEL M. PRESS, MD

Medical Director
Spine and Sports Rehabilitation
Rehabilitation Institute of Chicago

Associate Professor
Physical Medicine and Rehabilitation
Northwestern University Feinberg School of Medicine

President, North American Spine Society, 2005–2006

President, American Academy of
Physical Medicine and Rehabilitation, 2006–2007

Preface to the Second Edition

Mike Hage was a gifted clinician and teacher who had a unique ability to educate his patients in a way that empowered them to take control of their pain. He wrote this book in the early 1990s to give people a tool to use in the management of their pain in order to lessen its impact on their lives. He routinely used the book in his everyday care of patients, and we continue to do the same in our own clinical practices.

This book has stood the test of time. Since it was first published, the book has sold many thousands of copies and has been translated into numerous languages. The information and advice that Mike wrote almost fifteen years ago remain the gold standard for neck and back care. In updating Mike's work, we made changes that reflect current physical therapy practice. We think these additions are logical extensions of Mike's ideas and embrace his original concepts while preserving the user-friendly and easy-to-read style of the original text.

All of us had the opportunity to know Mike Hage as a friend, colleague, and mentor. We are honored to have had the opportunity to work on this project, which will carry on Mike's legacy of excellent clinical care, teaching, and mentoring.

JO FASEN

SHARON FELDMANN

BILL KEELEY

ANNIE O'CONNOR

VIRGINIA WIRTH-PATTULLO

ABOUT THE AUTHORS

ABOUT MIKE HAGE

Mike Hage, MS PT, former Physical Therapy Supervisor in the Pain Program at the Rehabilitation Institute of Chicago, was working in the Spine and Sports Rehabilitation Center at the time of his death. He was also on the faculty of the Northwestern University Physical Therapy Program and he managed a small private practice. His teaching specialty areas included evaluation and treatment of musculoskeletal problems of the spine, the extremities, and the Temporal Mandibular joints. This self-help guide was the fulfillment of Mike's wish to return control to the person in pain, as that was the most rewarding aspect of his clinical practice as a physical therapist.

Acknowledgments

To my colleagues at Physical Therapy, Ltd., Northwestern University Programs in Physical Therapy, the Rehabilitation Institute of Chicago, the Rusk Rehabilitation Center (Missouri), and the University of Missouri Physical Therapy School: thank you for my professional life, my work, and the body of knowledge we share. A special thank you to those physical therapists past and present whose contributions to the field are obviously integrated within this text.

To my patients, who have challenged me with their questions, motivated me with their potential for improvement, and taught me to appreciate efficient, pain-free movement.

And finally, most importantly, to Annette and Maury Light—who made this all happen.

—MIKE HAGE
(from original edition)

ABOUT THE REVISION AUTHORS

JO FASEN, **MPT, OCS, CSCS,** is Clinical Manager of the Spine, Sport and Rehabilitation and Chronic Pain Programs at the Rehabilitation Institute of Chicago. She received her master's degree in physical therapy from Northwestern University Medical School, is certified in Strength and Conditioning, and is an American Physical Therapy Association Board Certified Orthopaedic Clinical Specialist. Her treatment emphases are Spine and Sports Orthopaedics, and general musculoskeletal injuries and pain, with a focus on functional diagnostics and treatment. Jo has published articles and research. She worked with the Olympians during the 2002 Salt Lake City Winter Olympic Games.

SHARON FELDMANN, **PT, MS, OCS,** has worked at the Rehabilitation Institute of Chicago (RIC) since 1989. She started out as a staff physical therapist on the outpatient team specializing in chronic musculoskeletal dysfunction and arthritis, and is currently the Clinical Manager of RIC's multidisciplinary Arthritis Center. Sharon earned her physical therapy degree from Northwestern University School of Medicine, and her master's degree in exercise physiology from Benedictine University. She is an American Physical Therapy Association Board Certified Othopaedic Clinical Specialist.

BILL KEELEY, **PT, MBA,** has worked in physical rehabilitation since 1982 and is currently the Executive Director of Outpatient Services at the Rehabilitation Institute of Chicago. Bill earned a Bachelor of Science degree in biology from Wagner College before pursuing a physical therapy degree from Northwestern University School of Medicine, and earning a master's in business administration from Loyola University of Chicago. He lectures nationally, treats both orthopaedic and neurological patients with musculoskeletal pain, and serves as a guest lecturer at Northwestern University Physical Therapy and Prosthetic and Orthotic programs.

ANNIE O'CONNOR, MS, PT, OCS, is Corporate Director of the Musculoskeletal Practice at the Rehabilitation Institute of Chicago (RIC). She has a master's degree in orthopaedic physical therapy, is an American Physical Therapy Association Board Certified Orthopaedic Clinical Specialist, and completed the McKenzie Mechanical Diagnosis and Treatment training. She treats both orthopaedic and neurological patients with musculoskeletal pain and has been instrumental in establishing Allied Health Core Competencies for Musculoskeletal Rehabilitation for the RIC. She lectures nationally for the American College of Sports Medicine, Physical Medicine, and Rehabilitation Conferences.

VIRGINIA WIRTH-PATTULLO, MS, PT, received her master of science degree from Northwestern University and specializes in musculoskeletal disorders of the spine, extremities, and the craniofacial region. A focus of her varied treatment approaches is to educate patients on managing their pain with self-treatment techniques/positions, and individualized exercises for their specific dysfunction. Virginia has taught in the Physical Therapy Programs at Northwestern and Midwestern Universities and has been published in the *APTA Journal.* She worked in the Chronic Pain Program at the Rehabilitation Institute of Chicago, which applies many of the treatments included in this book.

Introduction:
Taking Control of Your Pain

This book is a self-help guide for people who have neck or back pain. It provides a practical and balanced strategy for delivering self-care, for helping you redirect the way you move, position yourself, rest, and exercise. The major goal of the book is to improve your posture and body movement during your everyday activities so that you may decrease your pain and improve your efficiency and appearance.

You may be experiencing pain anywhere from your head, neck, and shoulders to your lower back and pelvis, as well as pain in your arms and legs that is actually coming from your neck or back. Your pain may have begun recently, or it may have been troubling you for many years. It may have started as a result of any combination of the following: an accident, degenerative structural changes due to aging, prolonged poor posture, repetitive movements, and/or an actual disease process. You may have been told that you'll just have to learn to live with it, or simply to stop being active. Regardless of the cause or location of your problem, or how long you have suffered from it, you can ease your pain and remain active in a constructive way by applying the good moves described in the following pages.

This book will not address specific medical diagnoses or the use of medications, surgery, and nutritional adjustments for various problems with the neck and lower back. Instead of providing information on how to diagnose and medically treat your problem, this book shows you how to take control of your problem through self-treatment. Its premise is that you can directly address any musculoskeletal problem of the spine by learning how to position and move yourself with better alignment, less effort, improved breathing habits, and a constructive outlook.

These are the good moves that will be described throughout this book. Your goal should be to incorporate these moves into every activity you perform, from driving to work to walking for exercise. This will take some concentration on your part and will require that you become conscious of your body's responses to various movements and postures. In order for you to achieve truly lasting pain relief, you have to be aware enough to recognize when you are performing bad moves (bad alignment, tension, poor breathing habits, and/or negative thoughts and emotions) and disciplined enough to replace these bad moves with the appropriate good moves. In this way you can stop being a victim of your pain and start taking control of your life.

How This Book Is Organized

Chapter 1 briefly describes your electrical and structural systems and explains how they are involved in decreasing or increasing your pain. What we are calling your electrical system is actually your nervous system, but thinking of this system in terms of electricity makes it easier to understand its role in carrying, storing, and interpreting both pain and comfort messages. This understanding will help you learn how to utilize "comfort circuits" to decrease your pain.

The structural system is the same as your musculoskeletal system. Regardless of your specific diagnosis, if your pain has been traced to structural problems of the spine, improving your ability to position, move, and strengthen your structural system will decrease your pain.

Chapter 2 focuses on those times when your immediate concern is pain relief. During short or extended periods when your pain has increased, you can use the methods described in this chapter to obtain quick relief. These methods include relief positions and movements, relief breathing and imagery, and use of relief "blankets" (heat, cold, vibration, corsets, etc.).

Chapter 3 spells out good moves and bad moves relative to sitting, standing, walking, bending, and lifting. If you learn to adopt some of the simple methods for improving your posture and body mechanics described in this chapter, you will certainly reduce wear and tear on your back and neck. The ultimate effect will be decreased pain, improved function, and a healthier, more attractive appearance.

Chapter 4 continues to describe good moves and bad moves relative to your daily activities. Patterned on the average person's 24-hour cycle, it addresses specific situations such as bathing, dressing, commuting, and doing housework, yard work, and office work.

Chapter 5 describes a strategic approach to exercise for individuals with back or neck pain. It clarifies why such individuals will benefit from improving their flexibility, strength, and endurance, and it describes safe methods for doing so. This chapter also warns you of bad moves to avoid while exercising; it steers you away from the wrong type of exercise and/or poor performance of exercises, which can aggravate your pain as much as total inactivity can. It is important for you to understand the quality of good, healthy exercise versus bad, stressful exercise.

How to Use This Book

Attempting to read through the entire book in sequence may be a bit overwhelming and may not be very efficient. The following recommendations are meant to help steer you directly to the information that may be the most important and beneficial to you.

■ Chapter 1 is short and provides the framework for using the rest of the book. It will be beneficial for everyone to read this first.

■ If you are currently in the midst of increased pain that limits your ability to perform daily activities, you should proceed directly to chapter 2. Read about the recommended relief positions and try the ones that seem to address your pain pattern. You'll find the breathing, imagery, and relief "blankets" sections useful no matter what your specific problem is.

■ If your pain increases or starts up as a result of specific positions or movements, refer directly to the related information contained in chapters 3 and 4. For example, if your pain seems to increase in sitting situations, go directly to the "Focus on Sitting" section contained in chapter 3 and to the specific sitting functions described in chapter 4.

■ It is very important that you feel comfortable with the strategies and methods presented in chapters 2, 3, and 4 before you get very involved with the exercise chapter (5). Many references are made in the earlier chapters to specific exercises contained in chapter 5. If you have questions or problems with specific exercises in chapter 5, refer back to these earlier references first to examine recommended good moves and bad moves.

■ At the back of the book there are blank pages for you to write out your own personalized program of self-care in quick-reference form. You may wish to include any or all of the following:

• list the positions or functions that you suspect most often aggravate your pain (see chapters 3, 4, and 5 for ideas);

• list the page numbers of the relief positions (see chapter 2) and postural recommendations (chapters 3 and 4) that are most closely related to your problem positions, movements, or functions;

• and/or make a list of the exercises that, according to their descriptions in chapter 5 as well as earlier recommendations, sound as if they may have a beneficial effect on you.

Getting Help/Helping Yourself

Anyone with back or neck pain could benefit from an evaluation and recommendations from a physical therapist and physician who specialize in the care of musculoskeletal problems of the spine. If you are currently under the care of a physical therapist, this book will provide you with an additional source of information regarding what you can do to help yourself, and the therapist will be able to direct you most efficiently to those recommendations that are most specific to your situation. If you have not seen a physical therapist or physician who specializes in back or neck care, then you should at least have an evaluation to determine the problem, to rule out other possible medical problems, and to learn about other medical and hands-on therapy approaches that might help you.

It is not necessary to undergo a medical examination prior to using the information contained in this book; however, it is important that you listen carefully to your body. If your symptoms do not respond to your attempts at relief, if they seem to recur, and/or if they seem to be getting worse, you are advised to seek medical attention.

There is no way to predict for you the level of relief you may achieve by following the recommendations presented in this book. You may achieve a quick or gradual reduction of the pain you are currently experiencing, or you may only achieve a minor reduction of your pain. In either case, becoming more active in your pursuit of comfort and your ability to function means gaining greater control over your pain and the effect it has on you.

AS STATED ABOVE, YOU ARE ADVISED TO SEEK THE GUIDANCE OF THE APPROPRIATE HEALTH PRACTITIONER FOR THE TREATMENT OF YOUR NECK OR BACK PAIN. IF YOU CHOOSE TO FOLLOW THE ADVICE PRESENTED IN THIS BOOK, YOU MUST ASSUME FULL RESPONSIBILITY.

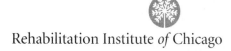
Rehabilitation Institute *of* Chicago

THE
Back
Pain
B O O K

R E V I S E D
2 N D
E D I T I O N

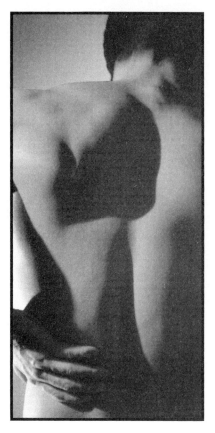

CHAPTER 1

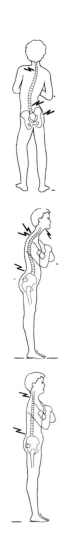

Your Electrical and Structural Systems

ⴸ

THE "ELECTRICAL" SYSTEM

THE "STRUCTURAL" SYSTEM

YOUR ELECTRICAL AND
STRUCTURAL SYSTEMS:
KEY CONCEPTS

Persistent or recurring pain is often the result of structural and electrical imbalances in the body. In order to relieve your pain, you must reduce these imbalances as much as possible. A good first step is to become aware of how these two systems affect your pain.

The "Electrical" System

Your "electrical" system is your nervous system. It is made up of all the nerves in the body, including the nerves of the brain and spinal cord. The electrical system forms a complex circuit that provides you with the power to automatically move, think, and feel. It also enables you to consciously direct how you move, what you think, and how you feel. Imbalance within the electrical system can result in pain, negative emotional and muscular tension, and fatigue. By learning to decrease some of these imbalances, you can increase your sense of comfort, relaxation, and energy. This can be accomplished if you take more conscious control of the following electrical functions:

Breathing

Your breathing pattern reflects the electrical activity of your nervous system. When you breathe in a rapid, shallow, or nervous manner (due to tension, apprehension, anger, concern, fear, stress, or fatigue), the electrical activity in your system tends to increase, and this can trigger pain circuits (Fig. 1.1). If you become more aware of how you're breathing, you can slow down your breathing and take fuller, more relaxed breaths (Fig. 1.2). This will lower the electrical sensitivity of your system and reduce your pain.

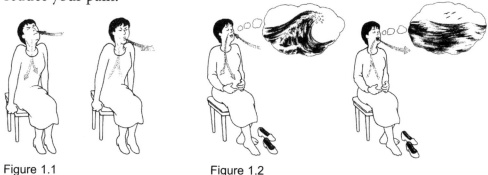

Figure 1.1   Figure 1.2

It is especially important to pay attention to your breathing when you are experiencing increased pain or stress. At these times, you may tend to focus on the pain or stress and automatically exhibit negative breathing patterns. Don't forget: controlling your breathing can reduce your discomfort! For more information on breathing see pages 31–35.

Thinking and Feeling

When you feel angry, anxious, tired, ill, or depressed, your brain automatically increases your sensitivity to pain. What would normally feel bad feels even worse. It's similar to the childhood experience of knowing that you are going to get punished—your fear can actually make you tense up, start hurting, and stop breathing before you are even punished. Your stress and anxiety can produce negative imagery, which only increases how much it hurts, how often it hurts, and how long the pain lasts! Focusing on positive thoughts and images while relaxing your breathing can decrease your pain, increase your

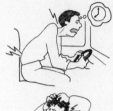

comfort, and help heal your problem.

Negative thoughts not only increase your sensitivity to pain; they also cause pain by increasing muscle tension. Feelings of concern, anger, or anxiety tend to increase muscle tension around the face and head and along the spine. This crams joints together and overworks your muscles, aggravating your pain (FIG. 1.3).

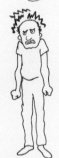

Feeling depressed often causes a slumped posture. Regardless of whether your depression is a result of your pain or some other problem, it is important to note that if being "down" emotionally means being "down" posturally, this adds painful compression and strain to your system (FIG. 1.4).

Imposing positive thoughts and feelings during your day (especially when you are seeking relief from pain, anxiety, stress, or depression) will help prevent your pain circuits from becoming overactive. The positive images help you to move your body into a less stressful, more attractive posture. The positive thoughts you use to generate positive feelings can be real or imaginary, and they can involve any people, places, or situations that help you to feel good, inside and out (FIG. 1.5).

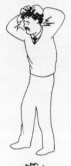

Figure 1.3

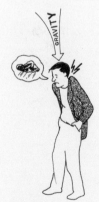

Figure 1.4

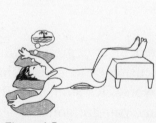

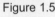

Figure 1.5

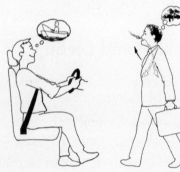

Muscle Tension

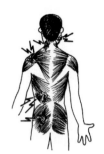

Excess muscle tension means that particular muscles are working too hard, for too long. This overwork creates a build-up of chemicals in the muscles, which often causes the formation of "trigger points," or "knots." These are areas of muscle that are extremely tender, tight, and contracted. Knots, trigger points, and muscle spasms are variations of the same thing—muscles contracting too much and too often. This commonly occurs in the jaw, the back of the neck, the shoulder area, and the lower back and buttocks (FIG. 1.6).

Figure 1.6

Excess muscle tension pulls and crams joints together. This increased compression can trigger pain circuits along the spine (FIG. 1.7), and this can cause increased pain not only in the neck and lower back but in the arms and legs as well. Therefore, it is important for you to become aware of the thoughts, postures, and situations that cause increased muscle tension. Then you can consciously control your breathing, thoughts, and feelings in such a way as to release muscle tension. This will lower the electrical activity in the region, release the tense pattern, and thereby decrease your pain (FIG. 1.8).

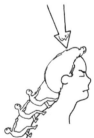
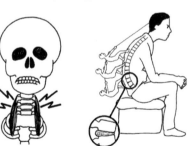
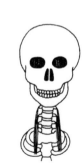

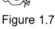
Figure 1.7

Figure 1.8

As noted in the preceding section, slumping also causes compression of spinal joints. In addition, sustained slumping can cause excess muscle tension by overstretching muscles and other soft tissues. When this happens, electrical circuits in the overstretched area attempt to warn you of the problem by activating pain nerves (FIG. 1.9). It's similar to slowly stretching your index finger back as far as it will go without causing any immediate pain. Within a moment or so, you begin to get pain messages—your electrical system is trying to tell you that damage may occur unless you bring the tissue back into more normal alignment.

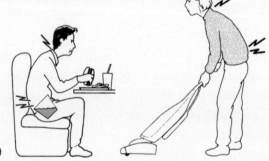

Figure 1.9

Become aware of your postural habits during predictable periods, positions, moods, and activities, and take note of how your postures affect your pain. Then you can reposition and support yourself to improve your structural and electrical balance, which will decrease your pain (FIG. 1.10).

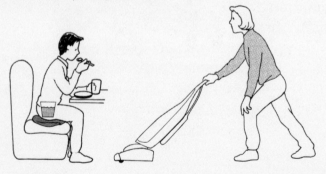

Figure 1.10

Tissue Sensitivity

A common reaction to long-lasting pain is to avoid moving, being touched, or doing things that you once enjoyed (FIG. 1.11) because activity in general seems to increase your pain. However, if you continue to avoid activity over a long period of time, your electrical system will become more and more sensitive, and this will make it easier to set off your pain.

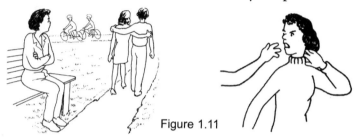

Figure 1.11

Your electrical system includes comfort circuits as well as pain circuits. If you totally avoid many of the activities you once enjoyed, your electrical system has no opportunity to use its normal comfort circuits. Hence, over time your electrical system fires comfort circuits less frequently, eventually firing more pain circuits than comfort circuits. Avoiding the activities you enjoy only increases your pain!

By gradually introducing sensations and activities that bring comfort, enjoyment, and pleasure, you can begin to allow your electrical system to fire its comfort circuits. Activities such as slow, relaxed, rhythmic movement, and sensations such as massage, vibration, heat, cold, and electrical stimulation (at comfortable levels) can all be used to boost the activity of your comfort circuits. Over time you can reprogram your electrical system so that you can tolerate more and more sensation. As your comfort level improves, you can increase your activity level.

THE "STRUCTURAL" SYSTEM

The structural system is your musculoskeletal system, which makes up the "mechanical" aspect of your body. It includes the bones and joints that make up the skeleton; the multilayered muscular tissues that connect, shape, and move the skeleton; and the various types of tissues that separate, cushion, and connect the skeletal and muscular tissues.

Many people have some kind of problem with some part of the spine's structure. These problems are the ones most often identified as the source of pain in the structural system. They may be caused by an accident, aging, overuse or misuse of the structural system, and/or disease. However, these problems do not mean you should have pain, nor do they mean you cannot perform the activities you enjoy.

Structural imbalances can cause or aggravate your pain. These imbalances may involve various stressful patterns of alignment and movement (posture) during daily activities, including rest, work, and exercise (FIG. 1.12).

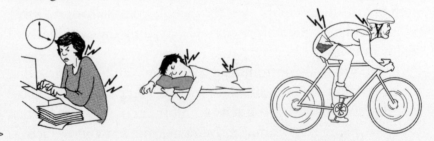

Figure 1.12

Alignment and Movement: Correct Patterns

Ideally, the spine should be straight and equally balanced from left to right. It should also exhibit mild curvatures from front to back, producing cervical, thoracic, and lumbar curves (FIG. 1.13). When the spine demonstrates this structural balance, the legs and arms are used most efficiently.

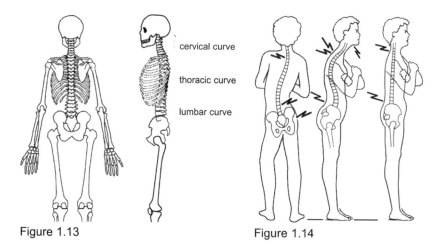

cervical curve

thoracic curve

lumbar curve

Figure 1.13   Figure 1.14

If the spine is not balanced from left to right, or if there are marked increases or decreases in the natural curves from front to back, increased wear and tear to the spine and other joints will result. This will increase the electrical activity in the pain circuits (FIG. 1.14).

Balancing your alignment and movement habits will not only improve your efficiency and appearance; it may also decrease your pain. In general, achieving such balance will involve the following:

■ exhibiting better posture during your everyday activities, especially those activities or positions that tend to aggravate your pain symptoms (see chapters 4 and 5).

■ avoiding doing exercises or daily activities in such a way that you add negative stress to your system. By being in poor alignment, cramming joints together, straining, and/or holding your breath, you are producing pain, not gain (see chapters 4 and 5).

■ exercising in such a way that you move and relax yourself into a more balanced state. This will generally include methods of decompressing, lengthening, strengthening, and relaxing (see chapter 5).

YOUR ELECTRICAL AND STRUCTURAL SYSTEMS: KEY CONCEPTS

Several important concepts have been introduced in this chapter. Since these concepts are referred to throughout the remainder of the book, you may want to review them before reading further.

electrical system: a simple way of looking at your nervous system. The electrical system includes your brain, spinal cord, and all the nerves in your body, including the comfort circuits and the pain circuits. Functions of the electrical system include breathing, thinking, and feeling.

pain circuits: electrical circuits that carry pain messages in the body. These circuits can be set off by negative thoughts and breathing patterns, poor posture and body mechanics, too much or too little activity, and trauma or injury.

comfort circuits: electrical circuits that carry comfort messages in the body. These circuits can be set off by positive thoughts and breathing patterns, good posture and body mechanics, use of relief "blankets," and balanced activity and rest cycles.

structural system: a simple way of looking at your musculoskeletal system. Your structural system includes your skeleton, muscles, tendons, ligaments, etc. Functions controlled by the structural system include posture and body movement during activity, rest, and exercise.

structural balance: refers to good, symmetrical posture that has a balance of alignment, strength, flexibility, and endurance. If balanced from front to back and side to side, the structure requires minimal use of muscle energy to maintain itself.

structural imbalance: refers to poor, asymmetrical posture that exhibits imbalances of alignment, strength, flexibility, and endurance. The imbalanced structure requires increased muscle tension to maintain itself and suffers greater wear and tear.

compression: describes the pressure of gravity on the body's structural system. The forces of gravity are increased due to poor posture and/or muscle tension, both of which can be aggravated by cold, pain, anger, stress, or depression. Over time, high levels of compression can cause increased wear and tear on the structural system, making it more vulnerable to injury and pain.

decompression: describes the reduction of pressure on the body's structural system. Compression is reduced by good posture and relaxed muscles. When pain has increased due to your being up too long and doing too much, use of recumbent relief positions (see chapter 3) assists with decompression of the spine and pain relief.

contraction: muscle activity creates tension known as a contraction. At rest, and in most stationary positions, there should be only relaxed, low-level contractions occurring to keep the body balanced and supported.

muscle tension: describes muscle activity that results in pain from compression or inflammation. This can be negatively influenced by poor posture, fatigue, and/or negative thoughts and emotions.

muscle tone: describes normal muscle activity in a balanced structural and electrical system during activity and rest.

CHAPTER 2

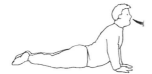

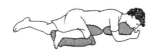

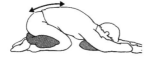

Quick Pain Relief

ᐯ

SEEK POSITIONS AND MOVEMENTS THAT RELIEVE

BREATHE AND IMAGINE RELIEF

USE RELIEF "BLANKETS"

This chapter describes methods of self-treatment for those times when you want pain relief, and you want it now! Whether you are at home, at work, or in transit, you can use safe, easy treatment methods to relieve your pain quickly. In taking active control over your pain, you are making an important step in the right direction. As you become more capable of reducing your pain, you become more capable of improving your general performance.

Relieving your pain on an "as needed" basis not only provides relief when you want it most. It is also a start at reducing your structural and electrical imbalances, which will help you achieve more permanent pain relief. The following methods for seeking quick relief will be presented in detail:

■ Seek positions and movements that relieve.

■ Breathe and imagine relief.

■ Use relief "blankets."

SEEK POSITIONS AND MOVEMENTS THAT RELIEVE

You may find that certain positions and movements tend to increase pressure, strain, and tension and thus increase your pain. Similarly, certain positions and movements may "unload" your structural system and "quiet" the electrical activity in the painful area, resulting in relief and comfort. It is important that you develop awareness of which positions and movements aggravate your pain symptoms and which ones reduce stress and irritation.

This section will present examples of common relief positions and movements prescribed for individuals with spinal pain. The positions that will work best for you may differ from those illustrated here or from the ones that work for someone else. By experimenting with the various positions and assessing their results, you can determine which ones provide you with the best pain relief. When effective, a relief position should decrease your pain within 1–20 minutes.

If you have arm or leg pain that is coming from the spine, remember the following:

Good Signs
▲ reduced neck/back pain
▲ reduced arm/leg pain
▲ reduced arm/leg pain accompanied
by a small increase in neck/back pain

Bad Signs
▼ increased neck/back pain
▼ increased arm/leg pain
▼ decreased arm/leg pain that is accompanied
by increasing numbness

If you experience a bad sign, this may be an indication that you are using the wrong relief position, that you've been in the position too long, or that the position is too extreme. Adjust the position or move out of it—you might find another position or movement that will relieve your symptoms.

If any of the following relief positions aggravate your pain, especially arm or leg pain, discontinue them until you can seek help from a physical therapist.

Low Back Pain Aggravated by Positions or Activities That Tend to "Round Out"/ Compress the Lower Back

This typically occurs during or after sustained sitting, bending, or carrying objects that tend to pull you down into a rounded, slumped pattern (FIG. 2.1).

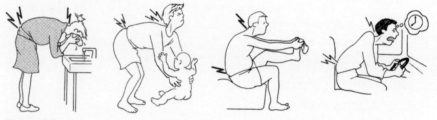

Figure 2.1

Relief Positions and Movements

These positions and movements structurally lengthen and decompress the spine. They will assist your body in "undoing" some of the compressive, shortening, and rounding effects that gravity has on your posture. Incorporate the breathing techniques mentioned on pages 32–35 in these positions.

BACK LYING EXTENSION REST POSITION (FIG. 2.2): Stretch out on your back with your legs resting out or up on a few pillows or on top of an ottoman, chair seat, or couch; try placing a folded sheet under your low, middle, or upper back to support your normal arch and to assist in lengthening the spine; by placing your arms up and out to the sides, you'll get a nice lengthening and decompression to your spine and chest wall. If your arms are tight, start with them supported comfortably on pillows.

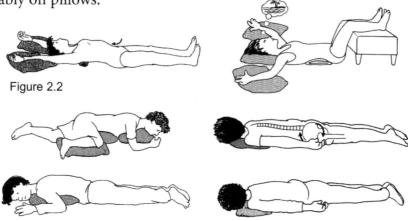

Figure 2.2

Figure 2.3

STOMACH LYING (FIG. 2.3): Place a flat pillow under your upper chest to allow your head/neck to relax forward on your hands, or to be turned sideways without straining. If you feel that lying on your stomach causes an uncomfortable amount of pressure to your lower back, place a pillow under your lower abdomen—this may be more comfortable at first, especially if you are not used to lying on your stomach. You may also find it comfortable, in this position, to bend a leg and place a pillow under it.

STOMACH LYING ON ELBOWS (FIG. 2.4): Gently shift your shoulders from side to side in this position; allow your lower back to relax and sag. If this position is uncomfortable for your shoulders, place a few firm pillows under your chest to

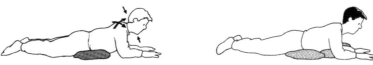

Figure 2.4

relieve some of the pressure. Relax in this position as long as it is comfortable. If you find this helpful, get into the habit of using this position in the evening as a short-term alternative to sitting.

PRESSUPS (FIG. 2.5): See p. 148.

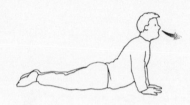

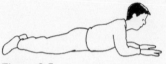

Figure 2.5

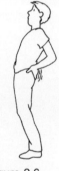

Figure 2.6

STANDING BACKWARD BENDING (FIG. 2.6): This move should be your first line of defense when you first stand up after sustained sitting! This is especially important if you have difficulty and/or pain when attempting to stand up after sitting awhile. Place your hands on your lower back and buttocks and slowly, gently lean back with your legs straight; don't tilt your head back. Stop when you feel a comfortable amount of pressure in the center of your back or across your lower back. Pause there for 2–5 seconds and take a Calming Breath (see pp. 32–33). Repeat 2–3 times.

SITTING LAID BACK AND UP (FIG. 2.7): When you can't or don't want to get up, recline and stretch out in your seat (see p. 54).

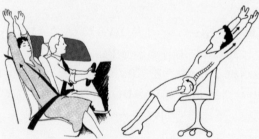

Figure 2.7

OVERHEAD BAR LENGTHENING/BACKWARD BENDING
(FIG. 2.8): See pp. 161–162.

WALKING (FIG. 2.9): Often, walking is the best way to relieve
low back and/or leg pain that comes on after sitting too long or
bending too much. See the "Focus on Walking" section of chapter 3 for tips on how to improve your form.

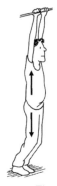

Figure 2.8

DESK TOP RESTING (FIG. 2.10): This method is especially
good when your symptoms have come from sitting too long at
a table or desk and you can't or don't want to take the time to
get up. Start out by pushing your chair back from the desk, then
gently arch your lower back and stick your buttocks out. If possible, spread your legs wide apart with your knees bent. Rest
your arms and head on the desk, allowing the spine to elongate
(sag) forward, and relax for about a minute.

See "Good Moves While Sitting" (pp. 52–63) for more
quick relief movements for low back pain brought on by sustained sitting.

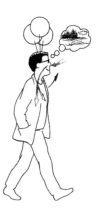

Figure 2.9

One-Sided Low Back or Leg Pain Aggravated by Positions or Activities That Tend to "Round Out"/Compress the Lower Back

Any of the methods just listed may provide relief here. By
adding some sideways or twisting movements to these positions, you may find more effective relief. Usually, moving the
upper and lower body away from the painful side provides relief. However, lengthening toward the painful side sometimes
works better.

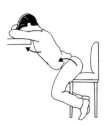

Figure 2.10

Relief Positions and Movements

SIDE LYING WITH TOWEL ROLL (FIG. 2.11): Lie on your side with the painful side up. Place a small, rolled-up towel under your side in the hollow between your pelvis and ribs. Place your top arm up and over your head. You should feel as though you're lengthening the top side between your chest and pelvis.

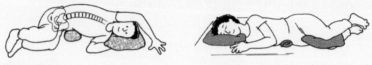

Figure 2.11

SPINAL COUNTER ROTATION (FIG. 2.12): Lie on your back and move your knees to each side, using pillows on the outside of the knees for more support. If resting with your legs off to a particular side seems to help, relax in that position for a few minutes, as long as your symptoms are decreasing (see pp. 142–145).

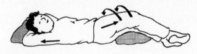

Figure 2.12

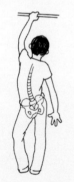

Figure 2.13

STANDING SIDE BENDING (FIG. 2.13): Typically, taking the weight off and lengthening the painful side is the most effective. By raising your arm over your head and bending away from the painful side (don't bend forward), you'll reduce compression. Use an overhead bar to reduce compression even further.

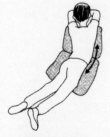

Figure 2.14

STOMACH LYING WITH SIDE BENDING (FIG. 2.14): This is the same position as the one illustrated in Figure 2.3, except that now you are positioned so that one side (right or left) is lengthened slightly while the opposite side is shortened.

Low Back Pain Aggravated by Positions or Activities That Overarch the Lower Back

This typically occurs during activities that involve standing, walking (especially when wearing boots or high heels), reaching overhead, or lying straight out on one's stomach or back too much, too long, or too often. Bad form while in these positions tends to pull the lower back into an overarched pattern (FIG. 2.15).

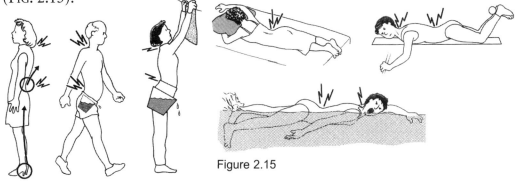

Figure 2.15

Relief Positions and Movements

These positions and movements serve to "loosen up" the lower back, enabling it to return to a forward-bending direction after sustained periods of being relatively arched (backward bent).

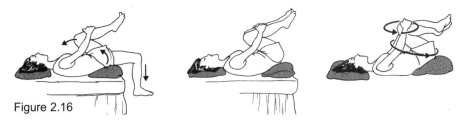

Figure 2.16

KNEES TO CHEST (FIG. 2.16): See pp. 146–148.

STOMACH LYING FLEXION (FIG. 2.17): This position is especially useful when you want to get direct pressure off your back. Place a pillow under your abdomen so that you feel a gentle, comfortable flattening of your lower back. You may find that placing another, perhaps flatter pillow under your upper chest will relieve any stress you feel to your neck. Yet another pillow under your shins and feet will add additional comfort. Similar relief can be achieved by kneeling and resting your upper body on the bed.

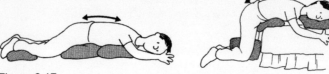

Figure 2.17

HANDS AND KNEES TO HEEL SITTING (FIG. 2.18): See pp. 149–151.

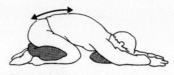

Figure 2.18

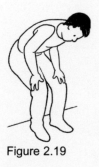

Figure 2.19

DECOMPRESSION SQUAT (FIG. 2.19): This is good when you need to get off your feet but can't. Brace yourself against a wall and move your feet wide apart and about one foot away from the wall. Squat down, making sure that you bend at the hips and knees so your rear end feels like it's sticking out. (Your buttocks should be leaning against the wall.) Place your hands on your thighs and take weight through them. By pushing through your arms, you can release the back muscles and minimize compression. Place your spine in the alignment that feels good to you— either mildly arched or rounded; just make sure you are taking the weight through your arms, not your spine.

COUNTERTOP RESTING (FIG. 2.20): This can be done over counters, window ledges, or sinks. Simply place your upper body and arms on a surface slightly lower than your chest and relax for a moment.

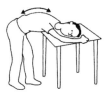

Figure 2.20

OVERHEAD BAR LENGTHENING/FORWARD BENDING (FIG. 2.21): See pp. 161–162.

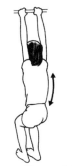

Figure 2.21

One-Sided Low Back or Leg Pain Aggravated by Positions or Activities That Overarch the Lower Back

Any of the methods just listed can be attempted. By adding some sideways or rotational movement to these positions, you may find more effective relief. Remember: movement of the upper and lower body away from the painful side usually provides relief, but lengthening toward the painful side sometimes works the best (FIG. 2.22).

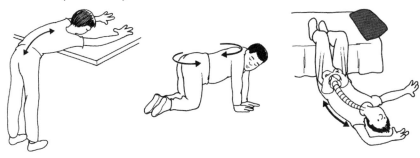

Figure 2.22

Neck/Arm Pain Originating from the Neck

The following positions/movements/situations tend to aggravate neck pain and/or arm pain that originates in the neck.

1.   Holding the Neck Too Long in Poor Alignment:

◆ FORWARD AND DOWN (FIG. 2.23):
  Xeroxing
  Typing, writing, reading
  Eating

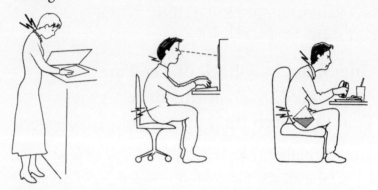

Figure 2.23

◆ FORWARD AND ARCHED BACKWARD (FIG. 2.24):
  Makeup/shaving
  Driving/poor visibility
  Bifocals
  Computer terminal too high
  Biking

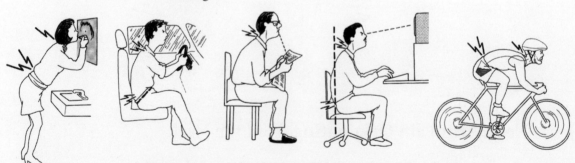

Figure 2.24

◆ Dropped forward and turned to one side (Fig. 2.25):
Looking out of passenger window
Computer terminal or document off to one side
Talking to someone seated next to you
Raking/sweeping

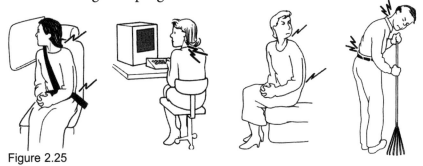

Figure 2.25

◆ Arched backward and turned (Fig. 2.26):
Unsupported stomach lying
Holding the phone between your ear and shoulder

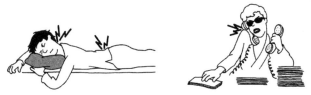

Figure 2.26

2. **Stressful Movements**

◆ Turning with the head forward and the chin out (Fig. 2.27):
Backing car up
Swimming—turning for air
Tennis

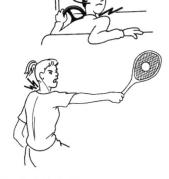

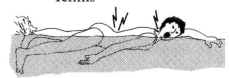

Figure 2.27

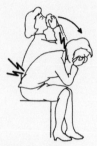

Figure 2.28

◆ Sneezing (Fig. 2.28)
◆ Tilting the head backward (Fig. 2.29):
    Drinking out of a bottle
    Looking up while cleaning, painting, lifting, etc.
    Lifting heavy objects

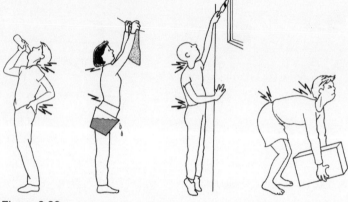

Figure 2.29

3.   Stressful Situations

◆ Cold/drafts (Fig. 2.30):
    Draft while sleeping
    Winter/cold and damp
    Swimming/cold water

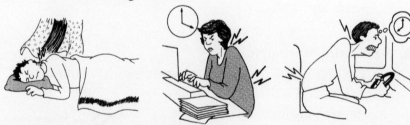

Figure 2.30   Figure 2.31

◆ Deadline pressure (Fig. 2.31):
    Office work
    Commuting

◆ ANGER/ANXIETY/DEPRESSION (FIG. 2.32)

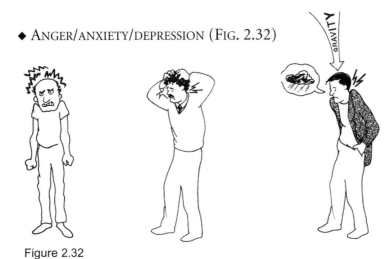

Figure 2.32

Relief Positions and Movements

NECK STRAIGHTENING AND DECOMPRESSION: This is one of the most important movements for you to learn for relief of your head, neck, and/or arm pain. It helps to balance your head on your neck and your neck on your upper body. It is especially recommended during and after activities that tend to draw your head and neck forward and tilt the head and upper neck backward.

It can be utilized for relief in all positions—standing, sitting, and back lying.

◆ *Standing:*
Glide your head back over your chest. Keep your eyes straight ahead. Keep your head level (do not look up or down, as this will tend to arch your neck back or bend it forward). Attempt to pull your head and chin back as far as possible without tensing up your shoulders or the

front of your neck or throat. Hold yourself in this exaggerated position while you consciously relax your breathing and muscles (FIG. 2.33). Rest in this position as long as comfort allows. Use your hands to help you achieve support and relaxation in this position. Repeat this move 3–5 times, several times a day.

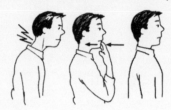

Figure 2.33

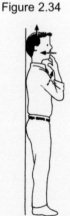

Figure 2.34

As you breathe, imagine your head floating up. Imagine there is air space between each vertebra—feel how this decreases the pressure on the pain nerves (FIG. 2.34).

While doing this exercise, make sure to keep your muscles light and relaxed! If you pull your neck in too strongly, you will tend to cause more pain. It should be a gentle, small movement of bringing the head back and in.

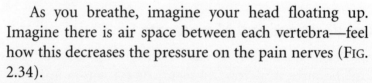

Figure 2.35

◆ *Standing—Using a Wall* (FIG. 2.35):

Stand with your feet about one foot away from the wall and let your upper back rest against the wall. Pull your head back with your chin tucked in so that your neck lengthens. Keep your neck muscles light and relaxed. This may take you 20 seconds to one minute.

◆ *Back Lying—With a Folded Towel:*

Make sure the towel assists in keeping your head level. If it is too low, your head and neck will feel arched backward. If it is too high, your head will be pushed forward (FIG. 2.36).

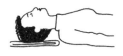
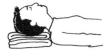
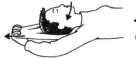
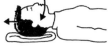

Figure 2.36   Figure 2.37

Once you are correctly positioned, reach back with both hands, keeping your head relaxed on the towel. Pull the towel so that your head and neck move with it into an even straighter, more lengthened position (FIG. 2.37). Relax in this position for a while and assess your results. Using heat or cold in this position may hasten your relief efforts.

◆ *Sitting* (FIG. 2.38):

See Pelvic Rocking and Head/Chest Floats under "Good Moves While Sitting," pp. 61–62. If you are in a chair with a neck rest, attempt to flatten your neck out against it. Push through your arms to assist in lifting your chest wall and moving your lower back away from the backrest as your head and neck glide back.

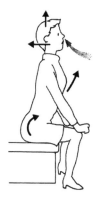

Figure 2.38

NECK RELEASES (FIG. 2.39): These moves are aimed at releasing built-up muscle tension and tissue tightness. (See pp. 137–142.)

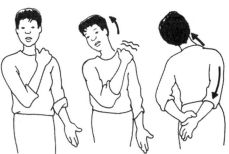

Figure 2.39

USE OF CONTOURED PILLOWS (FIG. 2.40): There are various types of these available from your local pharmacy, department store, or physical therapy department. The idea is to support the head and neck in its natural, neutral alignment. The trick is to find one that fits your dimensions and alignment. Contoured pillows can be very helpful in some cases, but the only way to find out how they work for you is to try them. (See pp. 128–129 for more specific information on contoured pillows.)

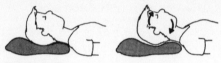

Figure 2.40

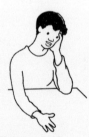

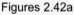

Figure 2.41

LYING ON TENNIS BALLS (FIG. 2.41): Place two tennis balls in a thick sock and tie the end of the sock so that the balls remain touching. Position them at the base of your skull just above your neck. Relax in this position for 5–15 minutes, taking occasional Cleansing Breaths (see p. 32). If the back of your head is tender, place a towel over the balls to provide a little more padding.

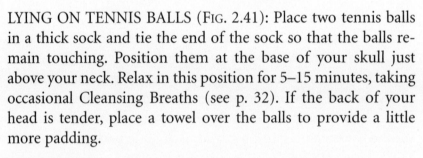

SUPPORTING YOUR HEAD IN YOUR HAND/HANDS OR AGAINST THE WALL: In various positions, this will usually provide relief. Experiment to find out which position provides you with the most relief. Usually, tilting or turning forward and slightly away from the painful side is the most effective for one-sided pain (FIG. 2.42a). If it hurts at the base of your skull and/or across the back of the head, try tucking in your chin, gently lowering your head, and supporting the weight of your head with your hand (FIG. 2.42b).

Figures 2.42a

Figures 2.42b

While employing any of the relief positions and movements described in this chapter, you should simultaneously use the following comfort-seeking strategies:

■ impose a relaxed breathing pattern,

■ visualize relief (this may simply involve imagining people, places, things, or events that make you feel relaxed, comfortable, happy, etc.),

■ possibly use various "relief blankets"—cold, heat, self-massage, vibration, supports, etc.—to help change the electrical signals to a more comfortable pattern.

BREATHE AND IMAGINE RELIEF

Your breathing is mostly automatic—you are not required to think about it. However, the way you breathe can have a significant effect on how you feel, so when you are in pain or upset, it can be helpful to take some active control over your breathing pattern.

Control your breathing so that it is slower and deeper; this may effectively reduce the intensity of your electrical pain circuits. Feelings of pain or stress may automatically cause a shallow, rapid breathing pattern, which often causes increased tension in the muscles along the throat, chest, and spine. This tends to compress painful structures together—ouch!

People tend to adopt a rapid, shallow breathing pattern when their bodies are in a "guarding state" against pain or stress. However, this guarding state actually makes you more sensitive to life's physical or mental stresses so that it takes less and less to set off your pain circuits! It puts the electrical system "on alert" and causes it to send painful messages even though no damage to the body is occurring. Imposing a relaxed breathing cycle (while in the relief position that works best for you) can help you balance the amount of electrical activity in your body so that the pain circuits have a chance to "calm down."

Breathing Styles to Impose During Periods of Increased Pain or Stress

Cleansing Breaths

Take in a long, slow breath through your nose. Imagine the air traveling to various areas within your chest, back, and especially your lower abdomen, filling and lifting those areas up with air. (Make sure you are not tensing up your neck, face, shoulders, or chest as you inhale.)

Pause for 1–2 seconds as you allow the electrical activity throughout your system to collect and build. Now . . .

Exhale through your relaxed, open mouth. Do not purse your lips or hold air in; let it gush out fully at any rate or force you feel is productive. Make it sound and feel pleasant. Think about getting rid of the "bad" air as it represents negative electrical activity in your system. Your lower abdomen should flatten again, assisting in complete exhalation.

Note: The in-and-out cycles should be easy, natural, and balanced so that you are relaxed and comfortable, not short of breath, feeling light-headed, or being concerned about breathing at the right time. Think of Cleansing Breaths as a controlled form of positive sighing that can decrease the level of activity in the pain circuits.

Calming Breaths

These are very similar to your normal, automatic breaths, but thinking about them will make them subtly different. For any few minutes that you are consciously controlling your breathing, the majority of breaths will be "calming" breaths interspersed with occasional "cleansing" breaths.

Calming Breath Technique: Inhale slowly through your nose, though not as deeply as during the Cleansing Breath.

Exhale through your mouth and/or nose and simultaneously think of releasing, relaxing, and letting go of the pain/tension/negative thoughts.

Thinking and Breathing for Comfort

For effective pain control and relaxation, combine specific thoughts and mental images with your breathing pattern during periods of increased pain or stress. Since both thoughts and breathing can dramatically affect your body's electrical system, they can have a significant effect on how you are feeling. By constructing various images in your mind's eye, you can directly affect the electrical activity in your system. By imagining/visualizing comfort, pleasure, and happiness, you can release natural chemicals that assist in blocking the pain circuits. Experiment with various images. Find those that help you to relax and calm the electrical pain circuits.

The following examples are common images that have worked for people taking control of their pain:

■ As you breathe, imagine an ocean wave in slow motion: as you inhale, the wave is swelling, peaking; as you exhale, the wave is lowering and spreading out, spilling cool water over your hot pain circuits, causing them to cool and calm down (Fig. 2.43).

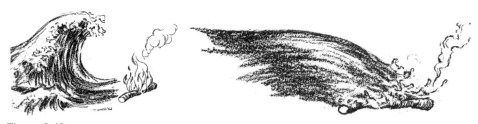

Figure 2.43

■ Imagine that your body or a specific area of pain is made up of a tight weave of fabric. Imagine that your current pain state is aggravated by the fact that your "pain wires" are being pinched and strangled by the tight weave of your "fabric." As you breathe, visualize how the weave spreads out and lets go a little every time you exhale. Allow this to continue—think of "release" as you exhale—and visualize how the relaxing of your "fabric" is causing less pressure, stress, and pain (FIG. 2.44).

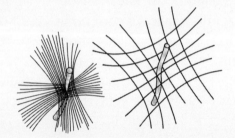

Figure 2.44

■ Imagine yourself in a place where you want to be. Block the painful area or sensation from your mind. Think about floating in the location and climate of your choice. Allow your breathing to keep you weightless. As you breathe in, feel your buoyancy—as you exhale, feel the pressure leaving you.

■ Pretend for a moment that you are feeling comfortable, happy, at peace. Imagine anything that would make you feel this way. Allow yourself to smile and be physically/emotionally "up" in appearance and spirit. Feel how a few Cleansing Breaths clear the circuits and restore a sense of comfort and well-being.

■ During periods when you feel weaker, more vulnerable, and tired, picture yourself in a Lucite cube. In this cube, you can breathe, move, see, hear—do every-thing you need to do—but the cube blocks out negative energy from other people or situations so that it simply can't get into your system. This allows you to be effi-cient, relaxed, and less vulnerable.

Repeat the positive thoughts and images over and over as you breathe—using both Cleansing and Calming Breaths while in the relief position of your choice. Beware/be aware of any tension that you are holding in any part of your body. Let your face reflect as much comfort and inner tranquility as possible. By imposing the outward and inward signs of comfort (posi-tive/relaxed face and body, breathing, and thoughts), you are confronting the reality of your pain with a constructive way of managing these difficult periods. Although pain is felt in your back or neck, it is perceived in your brain. By controlling the way you think and breathe, you can dramatically affect the way your brain perceives your pain symptoms.

USE RELIEF "BLANKETS"

Relief "blankets" may be used in conjunction with relief positions, movements, breathing, and imagery. They can be thought of as "that something extra" that seems to increase the effectiveness of your other, more basic pain-relief strategies. If your pain is not relieved by simply changing positions or ad-justing your posture, any one or a combination of the following relief "blankets" may be helpful:

- cold
- heat
- vibration
- self-massage
- binders, collars, and corsets

Cold

Use of cold has long been recommended for acute soft-tissue and joint conditions. Cold tends to "shut down" the blood supply close to the surface of the skin and therefore helps to decrease local inflammation/swelling. Cold can be extremely useful in providing some measure of pain relief, for it literally numbs the "angry" nerve endings in the painful area, thus slowing the activity of the pain circuits. Cold is especially helpful for pain that is concentrated in one specific area that is sensitive to touch and/or appears swollen or warm.

Cold should be used during the first 48 hours after an injury in which the skin is not broken. However, cold certainly can be very helpful long after this phase, especially at times when your pain seems to be worse due to too much activity.

If cold seems to help, use it consistently when you are using the relief positions that involve lying down on your stomach, back, or side.

Precautions

Some people react to cold (even in the form of an ice pack applied to a specific area) by tensing up. This negative reaction, if sustained, may actually aggravate your pain symptoms. Listen to your body. If you feel the cold is not helping or is actually irritating, do not use it!

If you have any problems with circulation, your heart, your lungs, decreased sensation, or open wounds, consult your physical therapist first before using cold.

If the area being treated begins to feel warm and stingy, remove the cold—continuing longer could result in frostbite!

If you seem sensitive to cold, avoid cold showers, cold drafts, and swimming in cold water. Oftentimes the cold can act as an irritant, increasing muscle tension and poor posture, and firing the pain circuits.

Methods

■ **Cold-gel pack/regular icepacks:** These are available in stores in various sizes; get the type that stay soft and flexible and simply keep them in your freezer until you are ready to use them. They will stay relatively cold for about 20–25 minutes. Use a light layer of toweling that has just been dampened with warm water. This will allow you a few moments to get used to the temperature before it turns cold.

Cover yourself up so that you are warm and in a comfortable position. Imagine that the cold pack is cooling down the hot pain circuits.

■ **Local ice massage:** This is most effective for smaller areas of muscle spasm or referred pain to the arms or legs. Hold an ice cube in a washcloth or cup to avoid freezing your fingers. Rub the ice gently in small circular patterns over the pain area or over the various trigger points illustrated in Figure 2.45 until the points being treated begin to feel numb, warm, and stingy. This usually occurs within 3–5 minutes, depending on the size of the area. Once this sensation is achieved, remove the ice and warm the area with a towel.

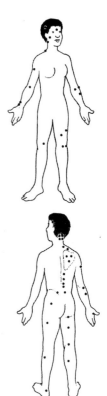

Figure 2.45

Heat

Gentle, soothing heat tends to stimulate the comfortable, relaxing circuits and may, in effect, decrease the "volume" of your pain circuits. Heat is also helpful in relieving muscle spasm, guarding, or tightness, thereby helping you become more flexible and relaxed. Heat will usually help if you feel cold, tense, or anxious.

Precautions

If there is swelling and increased warmth in the painful area, adding heat may aggravate the situation since it tends to cause increased blood flow to the surface tissues.

It is important to use adequate insulation (towels) between the skin and the heat source to prevent overheating or burns. If you have diminished feeling in the area, it is probably best to avoid using heat altogether.

Make sure you are lying down in a comfortable position with good support and alignment of the spine. Heat tends to cause the body to relax, so if you are not supported, the heat may cause you to slump.

If you feel warm, tired, weak, or depressed, heat may not give you the lift you need. Listen to your body and your moods to help you decide when and if heat can help you.

Methods

■ **Electric heating pads:** These can be shaped to fit the painful area and provide a quick and easy method for heat application. Some models produce a moist heat, which may help carry the heat to underlying tissues.

■ **Hydrocollator packs:** These are canvas packs that are filled with a silica gel substance; they are heated in water (160°F, 70°C) and will retain the heat for about 30 minutes. Use 6–10 layers of toweling between the pack and the skin to protect from burning.

■ **Microwave packs:** These gel-filled packs come in low back and neck models. Simply place the pack in the microwave for the designated period to provide adequate heating.

■ **Hot bath, whirlpool, sauna, steam bath:** All of these tend to result in a generalized relaxation response that may help to decrease muscle spasm and pain symptoms.

■ **Heat wraps:** These are commercially available and maintain a mild heat for up to 8-10 hours. This can promote a relaxation response, reducing muscle spasms and associated pain while allowing you to move at the same time. This is a safer alternative for heating while you are sleeping than an electric heating pad.

> CAUTION: BEFORE USING THESE HEAT OR COLD METHODS, CONSULT YOUR PHYSICAL THERAPIST OR DOCTOR IF YOU HAVE PROBLEMS WITH YOUR HEART, CIRCULATION, AND/OR LUNGS.

Vibrators/Shower Massagers/Whirlpool Jets

By sending your body vibratory, non-painful signals, you may balance and hopefully override the pain circuits. The vibration improves circulation and can greatly assist in muscle relaxation.

Use vibration when you feel that massage or gentle touch seems to decrease your level of discomfort. Conversely, when areas of discomfort are easily irritated by even light touch or pressure, these areas can be made less sensitive with gradual use of vibration.

Also use vibration when areas of discomfort feel very tense, thick, or in need of softening and loosening.

Methods

You will naturally do it right if it is feeling good and helping to alleviate your discomfort. If you find that the vibration is too intense and actually feels irritating to you, try insulating it with towels or your hand, or move it further away from the "target" area until it no longer feels irritating. Over a period of time, hopefully you will find that you can gradually increase the vibration without feeling so much irritation. When you can put more pressure on the area without the same uncomfortable sensation, you have made progress. In essence, you've taught your electrical system that gentle vibration can feel good! Keep at it—continue increasing the intensity of the stimulation gradually as the area becomes less sensitive. Combine the use of vibration with gentle stretching, relief breathing, and positive imagery.

■ **Shower massagers:** These can be directed onto areas of increased tension, tightness, and/or sensitivity.

■ **Hand-held vibrators:** These can be used on the back, neck, arms, or legs while you are supported in a comfortable position. Apply the vibrator to the trigger points illustrated in Figure 2.45.

■ **Whirlpool jets:** These can be directed to hypersensitive areas. Move far enough away from the jet so that the resulting stimulation is comfortable. Spend 1–2 minutes allowing the whirlpool jet to stimulate the bottoms of your feet—from the big toe to the heel. If this feels too intense at first, move your foot far enough away so that it feels good, and continue until you can tolerate the full force of vibration over your entire sole. Imagine your neck relaxing as the vibration is directed to the bottom of your big toe. Imagine your lower back relaxing as the vibration is directed to the bottom of your arch and heel areas . . . ahhh!

Self-Massage

Whether you use the pressure of your fingers, tennis balls, or other self-massage devices, make sure that it feels right. You are looking for a sensation that may not feel distinctly pleasurable but that makes you say, "Hey, this feels O.K.," or, better yet,

"This feels good—constructive, the right thing to do!" Adjust your techniques until you achieve this feeling.

Self-massage creates various forms of pressure that can assist in loosening and softening tissue and creating a relaxation response.

Methods

NECK ROUTINES:

♦ Push and pull the fingers of one hand across the soft tissues at the back of your neck. As you pull, slowly turn your face toward the arm that is pulling. Gently grasp and knead the tissues as you pull. As you push, turn away from the arm that is pushing (FIG. 2.46).

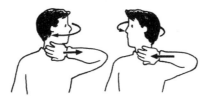

Figure 2.46

♦ Squeeze and knead the tops of your shoulders with one hand; support your massaging arm by cupping the elbow with the opposite hand. If you want to use both hands, sit forward with your back straight and your elbows propped on your knees (FIG. 2.47).

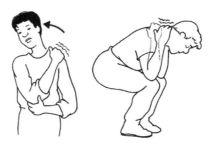

Figure 2.47

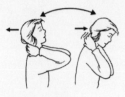

Figure 2.48a

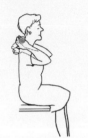

Figure 2.48b

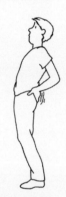

Figure 2.49a

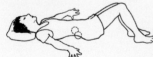

Figure 2.49b

◆ Slightly tilt your head back and place one or both hands in the small of your neck; sweep and massage the fingers together and/or downward as you lower the head forward and/or to either side (FIG. 2.48a).

◆ Find areas of the soft tissue in your neck and shoulders that feel tender and tight; use one or two fingers to apply pressure in a rhythmical fashion: clockwise, counterclockwise. An alternative to finger pressure is using a tennis ball to massage the area (FIG. 2.48b). Do not press so hard that you tense up from the discomfort. Imagine how your pressure is causing release of chemicals that can block your pain. Maintain relaxed breathing!

BACK ROUTINES:

◆ While slightly bending backward, grasp between your thumb and fingers the soft tissues on either side of your lower back and buttocks, and massage in a circular fashion (FIG. 2.49a).

◆ While sitting or lying, grasp and massage tense or tender areas. An alternative to finger pressure is to use a tennis ball to massage or lie on the area (FIG. 2.49b).

You will be more successful if you combine your comfort-seeking strategies. For example, as you practice self-massage ask yourself, "Am I breathing?" "How am I breathing?" "Am I thinking pain or am I thinking relief?" "Am I supported and at rest or am I holding myself in an uncomfortable position?" Get into a better position, breathe easily, massage gently, think about something positive, and get comfortable.

Corsets/Binders/Collars

These devices help to stabilize the painful area by "surrounding" it and limiting the amount of free motion. They can be very helpful in providing some relief for short periods of time, especially when you are up and about and feeling any of the following:

■ tired, unstable, and/or unable to maintain a balanced, upright posture,

■ afraid that the slightest movement will set off your pain symptoms (oftentimes sharp, stabbing pain),

■ unable to "hold yourself together" any longer than needed to continue functioning.

Wearing the support for short periods may enable you to be active when you choose and need to be while maintaining a relative sense of comfort and control.

Precautions

Supports can become aggravating if they put direct pressure over sensitive areas or if they prevent your body from moving and breathing.

Also, wearing the support too often or for too long can actually "de-program" your postural support system; if you overuse supports, your body can actually "forget" how to hold itself together efficiently. It is almost like the muscles know they have been replaced, so they go on strike. If this happens, your pain will typically increase when you remove the support.

Wearing a support is no replacement for rest in a relief position. If you have reached your limits, wearing a support should be second to resting; however, if you are unable to get into a relief position, wearing a support might be beneficial.

Methods

■ There is no magic in finding the right support—it is a matter of consulting with your therapist or doctor and of trial and error. If it is the right support and fits correctly, it should give you an almost immediate sense of relief by reducing the strain forces and allowing you to relax.

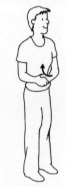

Figure 2.50

■ To help you prevent your own postural support system from "forgetting" how to hold itself together, you simply have to use your muscles within the corset or collar. For example, if you are using an abdominal binder to decrease pressure in the lower back, do not slouch in the support, expecting it to hold you up. Instead, feel what the support is attempting to do to your shape. Let your body assist naturally by thinking about how you feel more aligned; gently pull your lower abdomen up and in, away from the corset, while maintaining a relaxed breathing pattern. Look in the mirror more frequently to reinforce your upright and relaxed image (see FIG. 2.50; see Lower Abdominal Isometric, pp. 164–165).

■ If you are using a soft collar for your neck, be sure that you are not holding or being held by the support in an exaggerated or rigid position (e.g., with your head pushed forward or arched at the top so that the chin feels like it is sticking out). Take a moment now and then to gently straighten and decompress your neck (see pp. 140–142) and to move it in various directions—keeping your chin in as you turn. These methods can actually teach your postural support system how to "keep itself together" with less energy.

■ Avoid wearing the corset or collar for more than two hours consecutively without taking it off to assess how you feel: if it is continuing to help you, put it back on; if it is a relief to get it off, leave it off. If the corset or collar is helping, you should feel better, look better, and move better. If it is not helping you, then do not continue to wear it. It is essential that you consult with your physical therapist or doctor regarding your wearing habits, results, and questions. You must take the ultimate responsibility for deciding whether a support is helpful or not and for determining how and when you will use it.

Beware/Be Aware of the following tendencies and extremes when using the pain-relief techniques covered in this chapter:

■ Not using relief methods soon or often enough, perhaps because you simply don't want to bother or you feel inhibited by others. This only serves to reinforce the strength of the pain circuits.

■ Adopting postures and facial expressions that make it obvious you are in pain. This will not give you comfort; it is "pain behavior," and it is commonly unconsciously meant to evoke sympathy from others. It typically results in further aggravating your pain by causing more tension and compression and by focusing your attention on the pain circuits.

■ Using the "correct" relief position but not being aware of your general thoughts, emotional state, and level of muscle tension. If you are holding pain, anger, anxiety, and/or tension within your system, the relief positions will not be nearly as effective.

CHAPTER 3

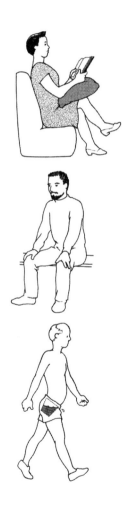

Good Moves/ Bad Moves During Daily Activities

ⱴ

FOCUS ON SITTING

FOCUS ON STANDING

FOCUS ON WALKING

FOCUS ON BENDING AND LIFTING

GOOD MOVES/BAD MOVES DURING DAILY ACTIVITIES: KEY CONCEPTS

This chapter describes steps in your daily activities that can significantly decrease the amount of physical work that is performed by your back. Simply becoming more aware of how you sit, stand, walk, bend and lift can improve your comfort, endurance, and ultimately the quality of your life. The following sections will explore bad moves to avoid, and good moves to incorporate into your daily routine.

Focus on Sitting

Sitting is one of the most stressful positions for your lower back and neck. Because of the amount of time most people spend sitting and the rarity of chairs that adequately support the pelvis and spine, it is important that you become aware of common bad moves and suggested good moves related to sitting.

Bad Moves While Sitting

▼ Slump Sitting (Fig. 3.1)

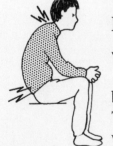

Figure 3.1

Slump sitting means habitually sitting with your lower back rounded and your tailbone rolled down and under you. This fairly universal pattern of sitting happens automatically when you sit on surfaces where the seat and/or backrest areas are too soft, too deep, too low, or concave shaped.

LET-GO TEST WHILE SITTING
Allow yourself to exaggerate slump sitting in the chair in which you are presently sitting: move yourself forward away from the

backrest and allow yourself to gradually let go of holding yourself up. Keep your head level but allow your pelvis and spine to slump onto the seat and backrest. While in this exaggerated pattern, become aware of the following reasons to avoid this bad move:

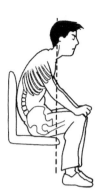

Figure 3.2

♦ *Slumped alignment*

First, imagine a side view of yourself (FIG. 3.2). Then, feel the location of your tailbone—it is probably down close to the seat surface; perhaps it has even rolled under you. Now check to see how the rest of your body is "stacked" above. Your lower back is relatively rounded out; your chest is "depressed" and may be practically "sitting" on your pelvis; your upper back is rounded forward, and keeping your head level now requires an abrupt backward arch at the top of your neck. Notice how your head is "hanging" or "sticking out" in front of your chest rather than being balanced above it. The more often you sit in this alignment, the more your body will become shaped and "glued" into this pattern.

♦ *Slumped breathing*

In this alignment your breathing becomes restricted and labored. Your diaphragm can't move efficiently and your ribs can't expand freely because the force of gravity is cramming your chest and pelvis together. Slump sitting produces a poor ventilation pattern, which can result in "the blahs," fatigue, listlessness, and difficulty concentrating. This alignment tends to shut the system down by interfering with the natural flow of energy.

♦ *Pain and damage to your structural system*

Slump sitting significantly increases compression and overstretching of the lower back and pelvis (FIG. 3.3). It is probably the chief culprit of low back pain, neck pain, and the degenerative structural changes that develop

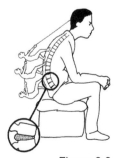

Figure 3.3

gradually over time. Pain may be felt in the lower back and/or neck; in more serious cases pain can also, or exclusively, be referred from the back or neck to the legs and/or arms. At times this pattern of sitting may feel comfortable, but it can actually result in pain and limitations while standing and walking. This is because the lower back has difficulty straightening up into the standing gear after sitting too long in a slumped, rounded pattern (FIG. 3.4).

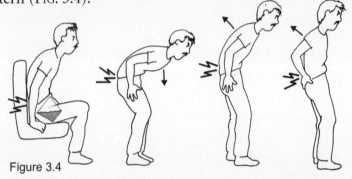

Figure 3.4

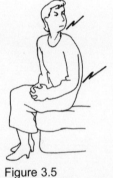

Figure 3.5

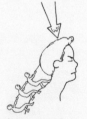

Figures 3.6

During slump sitting, the middle and upper joints of the neck tend to be crammed together because of the increased backward arching at the top. While slumping, slowly turn your head as far as you can toward one side, then the other. You may notice some strain or discomfort at the end of your range as the joints get crammed together in the area of the neck that is arched backward (FIG. 3.5). Because the head is hanging down or sticking out in front of the chest, the muscles of your neck and shoulders are overworked. The spinal joints at the base of the neck suffer a forward strain due to gravity (FIG. 3.6) As a result, headaches and various pain symptoms in the neck, head, shoulders, and arms are commonly aggravated by this sitting pattern.

▼ Uptight Sitting (Fɪɢ. 3.7)

Uptight sitting means expending continuous muscle energy to hold yourself up in a sitting position. It involves sustained, low-level tightening of muscles in response to unsupportive seating, stressful situations, and/or habit. For example, you may attempt to hold yourself up tall in soft, deep, unsupportive chairs by sitting forward, away from the backrest, and tensing up the muscles along the spine; you may hold your head and neck thrust forward to get through the morning rush hour; you may tense up various areas of the neck and shoulders when working under a deadline; or you may automatically tense the muscles of your face, abdomen, and rectum when sitting on the toilet.

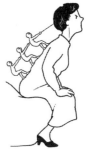

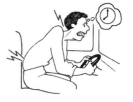

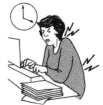

Beware/become aware of and avoid any tendency to do the following while sitting:

- ▼ Tighten up your forehead;
- ▼ Scrunch your eyes;
- ▼ Frown;
- ▼ Clench your teeth together;
- ▼ Hold tension in your neck, shoulders, lower back, abdomen, and buttocks; or
- ▼ Attempt to hold yourself up tall by pulling up with the muscles at the front and top of your neck and shoulders.

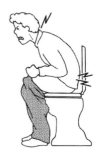

▼ Sitting Still Too Long

The human body is not designed to stay seated for very long without movement. The negative forces occurring during slump and uptight sitting will tend to shorten sitting tolerance even further. Even if you are sitting in more ideal sitting patterns, it is important to realize that the body needs periodically to change positions and move. It is more comfortable and healthier to move among several healthy sitting patterns that tend to balance the body with a minimum of effort and strain.

Figure 3.7

▼ Consistently Crossing Your Legs in a One-Sided Manner

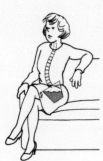

On the positive side, crossing your legs serves to stabilize your structure. This allows your muscles to relax, and, therefore it is often more comfortable. Crossing your legs tends to tip your pelvis to one side, which will produce a temporary sideways spinal curve, but this curve does not last unless (and this is the possible negative side) you tend to sit this way most of the time without switching sides. For example, if you typically tend to cross your left leg over the right leg, it shifts your pelvis to the right side, raises it up on the left, and causes your lower back to curve sideways (FIG. 3.8). Also, crossing your legs when sitting in soft, deep, unsupportive chairs or in a seat without a backrest will typically produce either slump or uptight sitting.

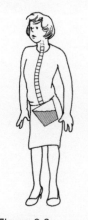

The solution is to become aware of whether you tend to cross either leg over the other consistently. After having your left leg crossed over your right for awhile, switch and cross the right one over the left. Switching your leg-crossing can help to cancel out the imbalance caused by consistently crossing your legs in a one-sided pattern. Also, make sure to reposition your pelvis (see below) firmly back against the backrest before crossing your leg—this will help keep you up in good alignment without effort.

Figure 3.8

Good Moves While Sitting

Whether you tend to slump or hold yourself tensely while sitting, the following good moves will assist you in achieving healthier and more comfortable sitting habits.

▲ Reposition Your Pelvis

This is a fairly subtle but crucial way to position your pelvis when you first sit down and to reposition it from time to time the longer you sit. The softer, deeper, and more concave the sitting surface, the more important it is to do this movement.

■ Place your hands on your thighs, armrests, or seat surface to help support you as you roll your pelvis and trunk up and forward into a comfortable, exaggerated upright posture. Now lift and lead your chest up and forward out over your hips with your tailbone sticking out behind you; do not allow your chest to drop or your back to round out (Fig. 3.9).

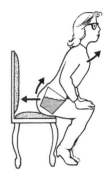

Figure 3.9

■ While taking some weight through your arms and feet, move your tailbone back as far as possible while maintaining a chest-up/tail-out posture. If you're in a chair with a backrest, arch your tailbone solidly up against the backrest. The softer the backrest, the firmer you should push your tail back up against it. Once your tail contacts the backrest, allow your buttocks/thighs to come down to the seat (Fig. 3.10).

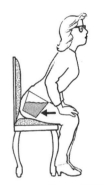

Figure 3.10

■ Now bring your trunk up. You should find that it is balanced in an upright posture with little to no effort. Allow yourself to let go—if your pelvis is adequately repositioned and supported, you should find that de-spite relaxing your muscles, you will remain sitting rela-tively tall and stable (Fig. 3.11). It's the difference be-tween being in "park" and in "neutral"—if you don't tilt your pelvis far enough forward to get it in "park," it will still be in "neutral" and it will roll back and down (tak-ing you with it) into a slumped position.

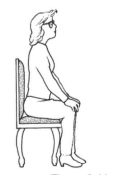

Figure 3.11

Note: Pelvic repositioning is the most important step—regardless of the sitting position you're in. In the beginning, or when you are in pain, it may help to exag-gerate this maneuver; after you have learned how to do it fairly automatically, it can be done very subtly. As al-ways, adjust this position so it feels good to you (this may mean rolling the pelvis more or less forward).

▲ Use a Variety of Good Sitting Positions

You should become familiar with a number of good sitting options that will allow you to change positions while keeping compression and strain forces relatively low. Notice that in all of these sitting positions the basic alignment of the pelvis, chest, and head does not change much; that is, the pelvis, chest, and head remain relatively parallel with each other whether you are sitting back, up, forward, or off to either side. What changes the most is the pelvic-hip angle (FIG. 3.12). The following good sitting positions are achieved by repositioning the pelvis and possibly using chair supports.

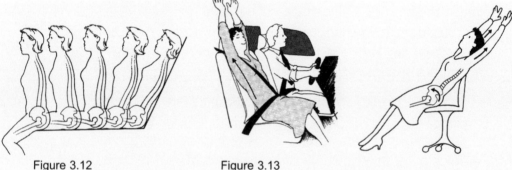

Figure 3.12   Figure 3.13

SITTING LAID BACK AND UP: Sitting laid back and up is the closest you can get to being horizontal without actually lying down. It can be great for reading, viewing, listening, and thinking. It relieves your lower back from the pressure of the backrest. Start by repositioning your pelvis on the front part of the seat in the manner shown in Figure 3.9. Then allow yourself to recline with your legs out fairly straight and your upper back/shoulders resting against the backrest (FIG. 3.13).

You are reclined in a fairly straight alignment that takes little energy to maintain and places little compression or strain on the lower back and neck. If the seat and/or backrest are soft, do not attempt this alignment.

SITTING BACK AND UP: Sitting back and up allows you to rest back while being active with your hands; it's a good alternative for those times when you're tired of sitting bent over your work. It is achieved in the same way as when Sitting Laid Back and Up, with one difference: instead of repositioning your pelvis on the front part of the seat, reposition your pelvis back against the backrest. This alternative can be used in virtually any chair that has a stable backrest (FIG. 3.14).

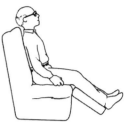

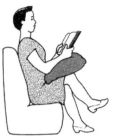

SITTING FORWARD AND UP: Sitting forward and up allows you to get closer . . . to better see, eat, and communicate. It also frees up the spine, relieving it of the direct pressure of the backrest. It's great for when your body is telling you to move your lower back away from the pressure of the backrest. It is achieved by exaggerating the Repositioning Your Pelvis move. Push with your arms and feet to lift and move your tailbone as far back and up as you can against the backrest before relaxing your buttocks down onto the seat. When you straighten up, you will find that your chest and head are upright although your lower back and trunk are balanced forward in front of the backrest. Take some weight through your arms on the armrests, the steering wheel, the table, or your thighs to further decompress the spine and support you up in this position (FIG. 3.15).

Figure 3.14

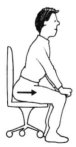
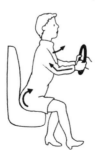
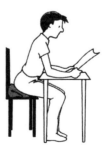

Figure 3.15

SITTING ON THE EDGE: This pattern is very similar to sitting forward and up except that instead of your tailbone being back against the backrest, you are toward the front edge of the seat. This alternative allows you to get as close as you want for writing, eating, talking, etc. It is useful when chairs are so deep that your feet don't easily reach the floor or when a chair is so soft, low, and deep that you may be "swallowed alive" if you attempt to sit back in it. Sitting on the edge involves repositioning the pelvis on the front quarter of the seat. Lowering your knees lower than your hips will help to keep you up tall. Moving the legs wide apart or positioning one up and one down will also help to keep you relaxed and stable. Your arms should provide some support—either on your thighs, on the chair, or on the table (FIG. 3.16).

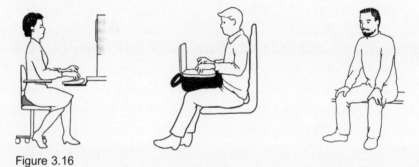

Figure 3.16

SITTING IN THE CAR: The design of most new vehicles attempts to address the issue of posture by providing mechanisms to make adjustments to the seat, backrest, and headrest. It is a good move to adjust the seat properly before driving.

Setting Adjustments for Car Seat (FIG. 3.17):

◆ *Seat Height*
   The best position is if hips are slightly higher than knees, as close to a chair position as possible.

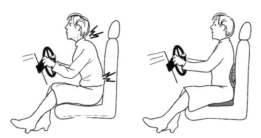

Figure 3.17

◆ *Seat Depth*

The best position is if your entire thigh is supported underneath you until just before the crease at the back of your knee. Move seat forward or backward so your knees are bent about 50-70 degrees; this position lessens tension on the sciatic nerve. This should also allow your elbows to be used at 90-degree angles so that your hands can move easily from the bottom to the top of the steering wheel.

◆ *Lumbar Support*

The best position is with your buttocks to the back of the seat, with the lumbar support inflated so that the spine is comfortably arched. Use the pelvic repositioning technique described on pp. 52–53, Figures 3.9-3.11, to assist in finding the right position and supporting it.

◆ *Headrest*

The best position is for the headrest height to be at the level of the back of the head and within two inches from the head. This may require moving the headrest forward or moving your head backward. This position can prevent whiplash in the event of a car crash.

If you are still uncomfortable, use towels, small pillows, or seat cushions as necessary to attain a better alignment.

In addition to attaining proper alignment, these additional strategies might help to make driving more comfortable:

◆ Make sure your jaw, neck, and shoulders remain relaxed.

◆ At stop lights, perform neck stretches and shoulder circles while using Cleansing and Calming Breaths.

◆ Use cruise control when safe and possible to reduce tension on legs.

◆ Take a 5–10 minute break every 1–2 hours. Walk and perform standing back bending exercises to restore lumbar curvature.

▲ Use Supports in Unsupportive Chairs

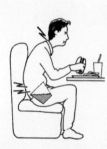

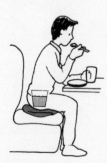

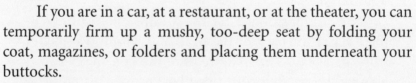

LEVELING THE SEAT: If the buttocks portion of the seat is too low, soft, or deep (relative to the front edge of the seat), your pelvis will tend to automatically roll backward and pull you down into a slump. By filling in "the hole" or firming up this part of the seat, you may immediately feel more comfortable and upright (FIG. 3.18). For relatively firmer seats (car, dining, office), put a folded sheet or two across the area of the seat where the back end of your buttocks rests. For extremely soft, low seats (couches, "poof" chairs), try placing a large, flat, firm pillow under you or a ⅛-inch piece of plywood under the seat cushion.

If you are in a car, at a restaurant, or at the theater, you can temporarily firm up a mushy, too-deep seat by folding your coat, magazines, or folders and placing them underneath your buttocks.

Figure 3.18

LUMBAR SUPPORTS: As the name implies, these are meant to support the low back region in order to preserve some of the natural curve (lordosis) that occurs in the standing position.

Therefore, the support should be tapered at the top and bottom so that it fits your spinal curve. The amount of curve stabilized by the support is based on comfort and the actual size and shape of your lumbar curve. Usually, the more lordosis you have while standing, the more comfortable you'll be preserving a larger lordosis while sitting, and vice versa; in other words, one size and shape does not fit everyone.

The particular size or shape of support you choose depends on the chair: the amount of support you find comfortable in a soft-cushioned chair will not necessarily be comfortable in a firm seat, and vice versa.

A lumbar support is only useful if you are sitting back against the backrest. Lumbar supports should also be considered secondary in importance to repositioning your pelvis and using a supportive seat surface. If you don't position your pelvis correctly, and if the seat is too soft, low, or concave, simply putting in a lumbar support will not address these primary problems.

Test the supportive quality of the chairs you sit in daily. Reposition your pelvis and allow yourself to let go. If the chair is the right shape and firmness for you, the seat and backrest will help to maintain you upright with minimal effort on your part. If relaxing your muscles causes your pelvis and chest to drop down easily into a slumped pattern, then more support is needed in the low back and/or seat areas.

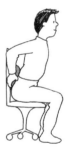

Figure 3.19

PROPER POSITIONING WITH THE LUMBAR SUPPORT: First, reposition your pelvis. Bend at the hips with your back straight and get your tail back against the backrest. Then lean forward at the hips, keeping your chest up and your back straight, and place the support behind your lower back and the top of the pelvis—if your tail is back against the backrest, the lumbar support should fit just above it (FIG. 3.19). Now straighten up and relax back against the support (FIG. 3.20). Assess it for

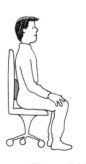

Figure 3.20

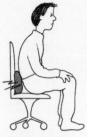

Figure 3.21

comfort, and reposition it if needed. If it begins to feel uncomfortable, take it out, reposition it, or get up and move!

Common problems with lumbar supports: With time and gravity, lumbar supports as well as their users will tend to move and settle. Most often the support will slide down behind you. If you don't reposition yourself and the support, it will actually encourage you to slide forward on the seat into a slumped position—the very position its use was intended to prevent! (FIG. 3.21) If a lumbar support is too large, you may feel uncomfortably arched in your low back area; or, again, you may simply slump in front of the support (FIG. 3.22).

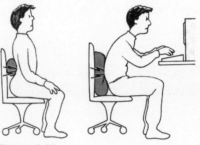

Figure 3.22

WHERE TO FIND LUMBAR SUPPORTS: There are numerous types of commercially available lumbar supports. These can be purchased at drugstores, in department stores, or over the internet. When possible, try out the support before buying it. Base your selection on comfort and the support's ability to help keep you up. When you make your purchase, have a specific chair in mind that you intend to use it in.

TEMPORARY LUMBAR SUPPORTS: When you're away from your home, car, or office, you can use various items as temporary lumbar supports. Try rolled-up magazines, newspapers, folded coats, sweaters, paperbacks, notebooks, comforters, airline pillows, etc.

A particularly useful temporary support is the pelvic wedge. This can be used in the Forward-and-Up and On-the-Edge positions. Simply take a folded sheet or whatever you are using for a lumbar support and place it under and behind your tailbone as you reposition your pelvis. This is similar to placing a wedge of wood under a car tire to keep it from rolling downhill (FIG. 3.23).

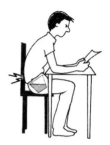

Arch up tall and try temporarily placing your hands under the rear portion of your buttocks in such a way that your pelvis is supported in a forward tilt—if you immediately feel more comfortable and upright, a pelvic wedge will help you. Make sure to relax your low back muscles—don't attempt to hold yourself in this posture with your muscles.

▲ Use Good Moves While in the Chair

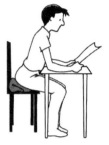

The longer you sit, the more your body will stiffen or tense and tend to take on the shape of the chair. By occasionally moving your body in opposite directions (e.g. standing up, performing back bending exercises, etc.) you will improve and preserve your comfort, mobility, and posture.

These moves should be used when you sit for long periods of time or whenever you are beginning to experience any sense of discomfort or slumping associated with sitting.

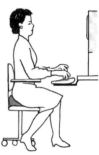

Figure 3.23

These movements are rather restorative; that is, they don't take much energy, they decrease strain on the body, and they assist in ventilation, relaxation, etc. Because of their nature they can be performed as frequently as desired. The actual motion can take 3–10 seconds and should be repeated a few times.

PELVIC ROCKING (FIG. 3.24): This is especially helpful if you experience any difficulty and/or pain when attempting to stand up after sitting too long. Rock your pelvis and lower back forward in the opposite direction from which gravity tends to

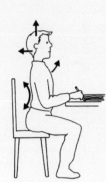

slump it: your tailbone should lift up off the seat, and the front of your pelvis will tip forward. Your lower back should gently arch forward to a degree that feels good to you. Use your arms to help take some of the weight off the pelvis and lower back as you tip them forward.

This motion can be done on the edge of the chair just prior to standing, or it can be done while sitting back, for example, while driving. Note: this is the same movement you performed as the first step in Pelvic Repositioning.

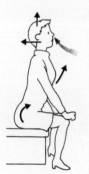

HEAD/CHEST FLOATS (FIG. 3.24): This motion can be done at the same time as you do Pelvic Rocking. It simply continues the natural motion that starts occurring up the spine when you rock the pelvis forward. As your chest lifts, your head will naturally lift and glide back over your chest. Gently assist and exaggerate this motion by encouraging the following:

Keep your eyes level and straight ahead. Looking up will arch the top of the neck; looking down will flex the low part of the neck forward. As you become taller in your seat, gently glide your chin back and in.

As you breathe in, allow the air to lift your chest wall and head; as you exhale, feel how they're "floating" up tall. Keep your neck muscles "light" and relaxed as you perform this movement. Your head should be floating up, back, and in, causing a lengthening and straightening to occur in the neck and upper back.

(For more good moves while sitting, see the relevant sections of chapter 4.)

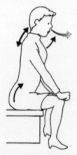

Figure 3.24

▲ Use Good Moves After Sitting for Long Periods (FIG. 3.25):

▲ Standing Backward Bending (see p. 18)

▲ Walking Tall (see "Focus on Walking" section of this chapter)

▲ Back Lying Extension Rest Position (see pp. 16–17)

▲ Stomach Lying (see p. 17)
▲ Stomach Lying on Elbows (see pp. 17–18)
▲ Swimming (see pp. 218–220)
▲ Overhead Bar Lengthening (see pp. 161–162)
▲ Cross-Country Skiing (see pp. 214–216)
▲ Lower Abdominal Isometric—Standing (see p. 165)

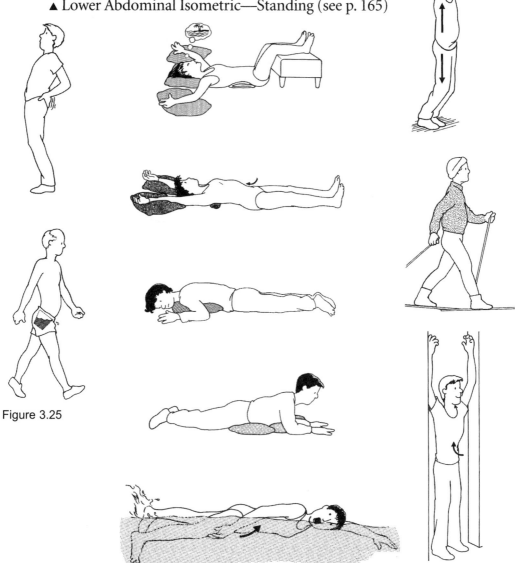

Figure 3.25

FOCUS ON STANDING

An important step toward standing more comfortably is to learn how to move and support your feet, legs, pelvis, and spine in more balanced alignments that reduce compression and strain on the body. Although each individual is unique with respect to his or her most efficient and comfortable posture, this section will present both specific and general recommendations that should assist you in making quick improvements in comfort, efficiency, and appearance.

Ideal standing postures support the body in relatively balanced, upright alignments with minimal use of muscle energy, and with no sense of strain to the body tissues. Occasional use of Cleansing Breaths and stretching while standing serve to improve alignment, release built-up tension, and reventilate your system. While standing, you should move about and use alternate postures in any way that feels good to you. This will improve your comfort and endurance.

It is most important to improve your awareness of your typical standing alignment and habits. By becoming more aware of your problem alignments and habits—what they look like and feel like—you will be able to decrease their frequency and intensity. As your alignment and postural habits improve, your structure will experience less stress and strain, and this should assist in alleviating your pain while standing.

Note: Only those postural imbalances that you can learn to control by moving or shifting will be considered. Postural imbalances due to leg-length differences, muscle spasm, or bony abnormality should be specifically assessed by a physical therapist or doctor. They will not be addressed here.

Let-Go Test While Standing

Stand with your side toward a full-length mirror. It's best if you can use two mirrors, placing them at an angle so that you can look fairly straight ahead while getting a side view of your-self (FIG. 3.26).

Take in a deep breath. As you exhale, allow yourself to re-lax; let go of any tense holding. Allow yourself to assume a pos-ture that feels like an exaggeration of your typical standing pos-ture at the end of a rough day. Visualize the major body areas as a series of blocks that are stacked up onto each other: one block each for the head, trunk, pelvis, and each knee and foot. Be-come aware of how your body "blocks" are stacked in relation to each other. Then check the alignment of your body "blocks" from the side and from the front.

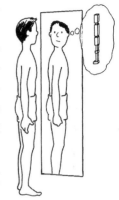

Figure 3.26

Side View

◆ CHECK YOUR KNEES.

a. Ideal—they should appear relaxed and relatively straight, but not locked (FIG. 3.27a).

b. Or, are they locked, or actually pushed backwards? (FIG. 3.27b)

c. Or, are they bent to an increased degree? (FIG. 3.27c)

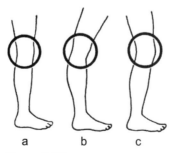

a   b   c

Figure 3.27

Note: If your knees appear to be locked or bent, move them so they are relatively straight without being locked. Notice whether this has an effect on which way your pelvis is tipped (forward or backward).

◆ CHECK YOUR LOWER BACK, ABDOMEN, AND PELVIS.

a. Ideal—there should be a mild forward curve in the contour of your lower back; your lower abdomen should appear flat and toned even when it's relaxed; if your pelvis were a bowl of water, it should be fairly level from front to back so that no water would tend to spill out (FIG. 3.28a).

b. Or, is the curve in your lower back increased, creating a definite forward arching? Does your abdomen stick out in front? Do your buttocks stick out behind you? Does your pelvic "bowl" tend to tip forward so that water would tend to spill out the front? (FIG. 3.28b)

c. Or, is there little to no forward curve in your lower back so that it appears flat, or even rounded? Do you tend to have a flat bottom? Does your pelvic bowl tip backward so that water would tend to spill out the back? (FIG. 3.28c)

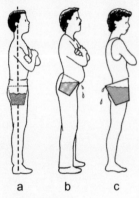

a   b   c

Figure 3.28

◆ CHECK YOUR TRUNK AND CHEST.

a. Ideal—the front of your chest should be fairly upright and relaxed; you should feel like there's some air space between the top of your pelvis and the bottom of your ribcage; the contour of your upper back should be fairly straight (or slightly rounded forward) so that your trunk is up tall (FIG. 3.29a).

b. Or, does your chest tend to be depressed so that your breastbone points toward the floor and your ribs tend to be compressed together? Does your chest wall appear to be practically "sitting" on your pelvis? Does the contour of your upper back appear to be definitely rounded forward so that you appear to be much shorter than you actually are? (Fig. 3.29b)

c. Or, do you tend to hold your chest up and out to an exaggerated degree? Do you tend to hold your shoulders up high by using your muscles? (Fig. 3.29c) If you think either of these are occurring, notice the effect your chest position may have on the position and tension of your lower back/pelvis and head/neck "blocks."

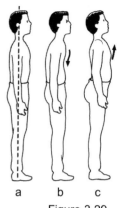

a   b   c

Figure 3.29

◆ Check your head and neck.

a. Ideal—your head should be level and fairly centered over the top of your chest; your neck should appear fairly straight with a slight forward curve; the muscles around the throat, the back of the neck, and the tops of the shoulders should appear relaxed (Fig. 3.30a).

b. Or, does your head appear to be "hanging" forward and down so that the base of the neck is bent forward? Do you tend to look down at the ground when you are standing still or walking? (Fig. 3.30b)

c. Or, does your head appear to be pushed or held forward so that your chin and/or throat are sticking out? Do the muscles around the throat and/or tops of the shoulders appear tight or tense? (Fig. 3.30c)

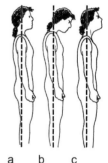

a   b   c

Figure 3.30

◆ Check the overall alignment among your head, chest, pelvis, and base of support (between your feet).

a. Ideal—your pelvis, chest, and head should be vertically balanced over each other and over your base of support (Fig. 3.31a).

b. Or, does your pelvis tend to sway out in front of your base of support so that your abdomen is sticking out in front (abdomen leading)? (FIG. 3.31b)

c. Or, do you tend to hold your chest up and out in front of your pelvis and base of support (chest leading)? (FIG. 3.31c)

d. Or, does your head tend to hang or stick out in front of your chest and pelvis (head leading)? (FIG. 3.31d)

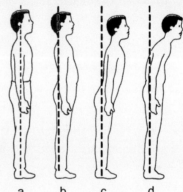

Figure 3.31   a   b   c   d

Front View

◆ CHECK YOUR BASE OF SUPPORT.

a. Ideal—your feet should be shoulder width to pelvic width apart; you should be able to imagine a fairly direct straight line from each foot through each knee to each hip (FIG. 3.32a).

b. Or, do you tend to keep your feet much closer together? (FIG. 3.32b) (This habit tends to increase muscle tension because the body has to work harder to maintain its balance.)

c. Or, when you stand in one spot, do your feet and knees tend to "splay" out to the sides? (FIG. 3.32c)

(This habit tends to strain ligaments in the feet and knees; there is no longer a direct line between the feet, knees, and hips.)

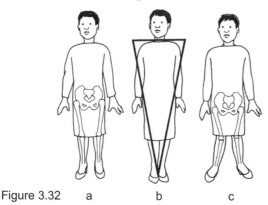

Figure 3.32   a   b   c

◆ CHECK YOUR TENDENCY TO SHIFT OFF ONTO ONE SIDE.

Shifting off onto one leg is a normal habit that serves to reduce muscle fatigue and compression (FIG. 3.33a). Become aware of any consistent tendency to shift your weight onto one particular leg. As with crossing your legs while sitting, if you habitually shift your weight to one side only, you're setting yourself up for alignment and strength imbalances. If you tend to shift off onto one particular leg, make sure to alternate sides—that is, if you are shifting onto the left leg for five minutes, follow up by shifting onto the right leg.

Also beware of habitually shifting too far onto one leg. For example, when you are shifted onto your left leg with your right leg forward, if you look down, you should see that the left side of your pelvis and your left hip are balanced over your left foot. If instead you see that the left side of your pelvis and hip are to the outside of your left foot, and that the right side of your pelvis is dropped, you are shifted too far (FIG. 3.33b).

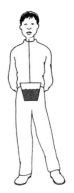

Figure 3.33a

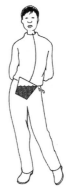

Figure 3.33b

Good Moves While Standing

▲ Postural Adjustment Exercises

These are simple, subtle shifts in the position and tone of your various body "blocks" that you perform while standing. They are intended momentarily to exaggerate improved alignment. As you repeatedly exaggerate improved alignment, your postural "computer" will begin to "store" this improved alignment as normal, and it will begin to occur more automatically.

▲ Structural Balancing Exercises

These exercises stress strengthening and lengthening and improved alignment. They are primarily done on the floor or bed. They are meant to assist in rebalancing soft tissues that are binding you or don't support you adequately or equally from front to back, or side to side. Recommendations on how to improve your specific standing habits through structural balancing exercises will be made in this chapter, but these exercises will be detailed in the first two sections of chapter 5.

▲ Improved Shoes or Inserts

These are meant to assist in supporting and cushioning your feet, legs, pelvis, and spine. Recommendations regarding footwear and how it can improve your standing will be made in the "Focus on Walking" section of this chapter.

Postural Adjustment Exercises

During these exercises you are exaggerating improved standing alignment. This will probably feel foreign and unnatural to you in the beginning. It is best to do these exercises for short periods of time (5–20 seconds) and frequently (3–5 times/day) until you feel that improved alignment is occurring more consistently and automatically.

It is most beneficial to adjust your standing posture with these exercises during those activities or times when you tend to exhibit poor posture. Attempt to perform your postural adjustment exercises during times when you are standing in one place—for example, morning and evening bathroom times, while waiting for elevators, while in line, etc. Keep the adjustment exercise easy and relaxed. Use Calming Breaths and the images recommended and perform the postural adjustment while watching yourself in a mirror (sideways). You should be able to see the improvement immediately. Allow the image of your "new" posture to sink into your mind's eye while you watch.

The following examples include some of the most common problem standing postures. Each example includes a recommended postural adjustment exercise to help minimize the problem immediately, and the appropriate structural rebalancing exercises are also listed. If you recognize any of the poor alignments as being similar to your own, perform the postural adjustment exercises as recommended. Ignore the postures and recommendations that do not look like your alignment.

Problem Posture:
Abdomen and Buttocks Sticking Out (Fig. 3.34)

a. This pelvic position causes the abdomen to stick out in front and the buttocks to stick out in back. This alignment is probably the chief cause of low back pain while standing.

b. Your pelvic bowl is tipped forward so that the water tends to spill out the front—this causes an increased arch in your lower back.

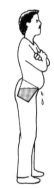

Figure 3.34

ADJUSTMENT EXERCISE: LEVEL THE PELVIS (Fig. 3.35)

a. Gently tilt your pelvic "bowl" so that the front "brim" moves up and under you—so that the water is level and tranquil (not held tensely).

b. Gently lift up and in with your lower abdominal muscles to help lift the front of the pelvis. Think of pulling your abdomen in away from the waistband of your pants. Allow your

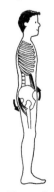

Figure 3.35

lower back to relax and lengthen into less of an arched pattern. Bring your tail down and under you by gently tensing the buttocks muscles.

Note: Do not pull the chest down toward the pelvis. Bring the front of your pelvis up under your upright chest. It is common to feel some minor low back discomfort when first attempting this adjustment. Make sure to keep the adjustment gentle, with a comfortable amount of muscle tension. Continue to breathe.

STRUCTURAL BALANCING EXERCISES:

- ◆ Knees to Chest (see pp. 146–148)
- ◆ Hands and Knees to Heel Sitting (see pp. 149–151)
- ◆ Hip Flexor Stretches (see pp. 159–161)
- ◆ Overhead Bar Lengthening (see pp. 161–162)
- ◆ Bridging (see pp. 178–181)
- ◆ Abdominal Strengthening (see pp. 163–173)
- ◆ Hands and Knees Reaching (see pp. 174–176)
- ◆ Stomach Lying Extension Strengthening (see pp. 176–177)
- ◆ Hamstring Strengthening (see pp. 194–195)

Problem Posture: Ostrich Standing (FIG. 3.36)

a. Knee joints are pushed back into a locked or even backward-bent position, forcing increased weight through the heels.

b. This knee position tends to cause the same pelvic and low back position described in the problem posture described above—tipped forward with increased low back arch.

c. Chest is depressed, "sitting" on the pelvis.

d. The head and neck will tend to drop forward and down, following the chest position.

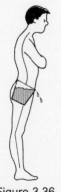

Figure 3.36

ADJUSTMENT EXERCISE: UNLOCK THE KNEES,
LEVEL THE PELVIS, HEAD/CHEST FLOAT (Fig. 3.37)

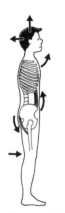

a. Unlock the knees: Relieve the backward strain and let your knees shift forward slightly, over the front of your ankles. This will be easier if you're wearing slight heels as opposed to flats.

b. Level the pelvis as described under the first problem posture described above.

c. Allow your chest to expand and lift with air as you breathe in; allow it to stay floating up tall over your level pelvis as you exhale.

Figure 3.37

d. Allow your head to float up tall and level, centered over your upright chest—as if it were filled with helium or being pulled upward by a string, with no effort on your part (see p. 62).

STRUCTURAL BALANCING EXERCISES:

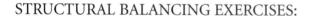

- ◆ Neck Straightening and Decompression (see pp. 27–29)
- ◆ Knees to Chest (see pp. 146–148)
- ◆ Hip Flexor Stretches (see pp. 159–161)
- ◆ Overhead Bar Lengthening (see pp. 161–162)
- ◆ Bridging (see pp. 178–181)
- ◆ Abdominal Strengthening (see pp. 163–173)
- ◆ Neck Strengthening (see pp. 173–174)
- ◆ Hands and Knees Reaching (see pp. 174–176)
- ◆ Stomach Lying Extension Strengthening (see pp. 176–177)
- ◆ Standing Leg Lift (see pp. 182–184)
- ◆ Hamstring Strengthening (see pp. 194–195)

Problem Posture: Slumping with Your Abdomen Leading Out over Your "Skis" (FIG. 3.38)

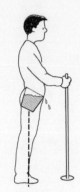

Figure 3.38

a. Your pelvis and abdomen are leaning out in front, forcing increased weight through the balls of the feet.

b. The upper body may compensate by slumping: chest "sitting" on the abdomen and head dropped down and forward.

ADJUSTMENT EXERCISE:
CENTERING THE PELVIS, HEAD/CHEST FLOAT (FIG. 3.39)

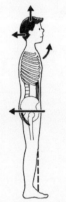

Figure 3.39

a. Bring your pelvis back, centering it over your base of support so that you feel increased weight through your heels.

b. Allow the chest and head to lift when you inhale and to stay floating up when you exhale. Imagine a string lifting you up tall and vertical, back over your heels.

c. Lift your lower abdomen up and in to help pull you back over your heels and lift you up tall.

STRUCTURAL BALANCING EXERCISES:

◆ Back Lying Extension Rest Position (see pp. 16–17)
◆ Neck Straightening and Decompression (see pp. 27–29)
◆ Spinal Counter Rotation (see pp. 142–146)
◆ Knees to Chest (see pp. 146–148)
◆ Overhead Bar Lengthening (see pp. 161–162)
◆ Straight Leg Raising (see p. 168–169)
◆ Bridging (see pp. 178–181)
◆ Abdominal Strengthening (see pp. 163–173)
◆ Neck Strengthening (see pp. 173–174)
◆ Hands and Knees Reaching (see pp. 174–176)
◆ Stomach Lying Extension Strengthening (see pp. 176–177)
◆ Back Extensor Strengthening (see p. 198–200)

Problem Alignment: Slump "Sitting" While Standing (FIG. 3.40)

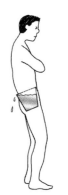

a. Your knees and ankles are bent excessively, as if you're getting ready to sit down.

b. Your pelvis is tipped back so that your tail is under you.

c. Your chest wall is slumped, "sitting" on your abdomen.

d. Your head and neck are dropped down and forward, following your chest.

Figure 3.40

ADJUSTMENT EXERCISE: STRAIGHTEN THE LEGS, HEAD/CHEST FLOAT (FIG. 3.41)

a. Imagine a string attached to the top of your head; allow it to pull your head up tall over your chest.

b. Allow the chest to lift up and to expand when you inhale; allow it to float up off the pelvis as you exhale (see p. 62).

c. Push your knees straighter, but not locked, and exaggerate a long, straight leg and trunk position—think tall!

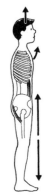

Figure 3.41

STRUCTURAL BALANCING EXERCISES:

- Back Lying Extension Rest Position (see pp. 16–17)
- Neck Straightening and Decompression (see pp. 27–29)
- Neck Release (see pp. 29–31)
- Spinal Counter Rotation (see pp. 142–146)
- Standing Hamstring Lengthening (see pp. 156–157)
- Calf Lengthening (see pp. 157–159)
- Overhead Bar Lengthening (see pp. 161–162)
- Bridging (see pp. 178–181)
- Lower Abdominal Isometric—Standing (see pp. 164–165)
- Neck Strengthening (see pp. 173–174)
- Hands and Knees Reaching (see pp. 174–176)

◆ Stomach Lying Extension Strengthening (see pp. 176–177)

◆ Standing Leg Lifts (see pp. 182–185)

◆ Back Extensor Strengthening (see p. 198–200)

More Good Moves to Stand By

▲ Prop, Shift, and Sway

a. Propping one foot up (inside a cabinet, on a box, on your other foot, etc.) and propping through your arms will help to level your pelvis and decrease strain on the spine (FIG. 3.42).

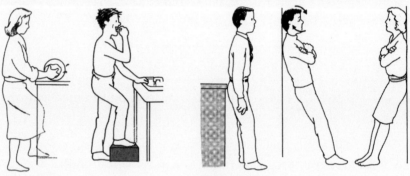

Figure 3.42   Figure 3.43

b. Leaning on walls, counters, poles, etc., will assist in supporting and decompressing the spine (FIG. 3.43).

c. Weight Shifting and Sway (FIG. 3.44): High-rise buildings have a sway factor built in to allow the building to dissipate strain from external forces, such as wind and gravity. Your approach to standing should also incorporate this basic concept. Subtle, slow, and small-range sway is a good way to relieve some of the cumulative strain of standing. Use of sway also assists in calming down the electrical system so that the muscles become less tense and the nerves are not so excitable.

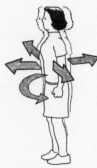

Figure 3.44

The patterns of sway are limitless. Do what feels most comfortable to you and be sure to stay in upright, relaxed alignments as you sway. Use any of the following sway patterns when you have to stand in place: sway from side to side; sway from front to back; rock back on heels/forward on toes.

▲ Seek Comfort After Standing Too Long

Use the relief positions and movements suggested for relief of low back pain that is aggravated by positions and activities that tend to overarch the lower back (see pp. 21–23).

Focus on Walking

Walking provides you with your most basic form of transportation. It is one of the safest and most effective ways to exercise the entire body. If your neck or back pain is currently aggravated by walking, your pain may be reduced if you control some of the factors addressed in this and the previous section (postural adjustment exercises). This section describes problem walking patterns (bad moves) and healthier walking patterns (good moves). It also makes suggestions regarding walking for exercise and improving your footwear.

Standing Reflects on Walking

In general, your standing posture will be similar to the posture you exhibit while walking. For example, if you exhibit an increased low back arch and/or forward-head posture while standing still, these imbalances will usually be present when you walk as well. If you tend to hold yourself tensely while standing still, your walking will also tend to reflect this tension. If you slump while standing, you will exhibit the same poor alignment when walking. Therefore, it is important for you to become aware of your postural tendencies and to follow the specific recommendations already made in the "Focus on Standing" section. Once you are able to make a subtle change to some of these tendencies while standing still (by performing postural adjustment exercises), it is a simple matter of continuing these and similar adjustments while walking.

If you recognize any of the problem walking patterns as being similar to your own, attempt the adjustments recommended. Use the postural adjustment, breathing, and imagery tips for short periods of time (10 seconds–1 minute) during your daily activities that include walking.

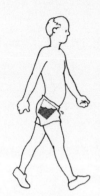

Figure 3.45

Replace Problem Walking Patterns with Healthier Walking Patterns

▼ Bad Move: Increased Low Back Arch While Walking (FIG. 3.45)

An increased forward arch of the lower back, along with a stretched-out lower abdomen, will cause the water in the pelvic basin to spill out the front as you walk. This alignment will typically aggravate low back pain. In this alignment, you tend to walk with your abdomen leading out in front.

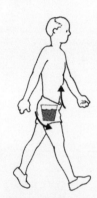

Figure 3.46

▲ Good Move: Leveling the Pelvis (FIG. 3.46)

(see pp. 71–72)

Imagine that there is a pulley attached to the front brim of your pelvis that goes up toward the ceiling. As you walk, imagine that the upward lift of this pulley is maintaining the front brim of your pelvis up and level with the back brim. The water in the pelvic bowl stays level from front to back. Allow this image to help maintain your pelvis and lower back in a stable position as you continue walking.

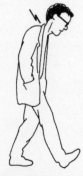

Figure 3.47

▼ Bad Move: Forward Head Walk (FIG. 3.47)

Looking down at the ground directly in front of you while walking will pull you into this alignment. This bad move may simply be a habit, but it will tend to become exaggerated whenever you are tired, ill, depressed, cold, or stressed.

A depressed chest often occurs along with a forward head alignment. The sternum, which is the front bone of the chest, is in a relatively lowered position. This results in poor ventilation and may result in decreased endurance.

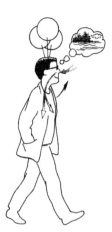

Figure 3.48

▲ Good Move: Head/Chest Float (FIG. 3.48)

(see p. 62)

While walking, occasionally take in a Cleansing Breath and feel how the air gently expands and lifts your chest up. Imagine that the air inside your lungs is helium. As you walk, feel how the air gently lifts the weight of your chest up and off your abdomen and pelvis. Allow your head to float up tall and level. Imagine that your head is a helium-filled balloon—feel how it can float up off the neck, and feel the decrease in muscle tension and compression around the neck.

▼ Bad Move: Floppy Walk (FIG. 3.49)

This walking tendency is characterized by wobbling and extraneous movements of various areas of your body. It generally occurs when there is a tendency for joint/muscle instability, which results in too much movement. This can result in pain in numerous areas, especially the neck, lower back, and pelvis. This type of walking pattern is usually associated with an increase in the spinal curves and a decrease in strength.

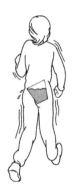

Figure 3.49

The water in the pelvic bowl is flopping around due to the tipping and tilting of these areas as you walk.

▲ Good Move: Impose Calm/Stable Walking
(FIG. 3.50)

Imagine that your pelvic and head bowls are ½–¾ full of water. Walk in such a way that the water stays relatively level and calm. Think of keeping the water "tranquil"—limit extra movement of the pelvis, and keep your head from tipping forward and/or off to the side as you stride. If you tighten up anywhere,

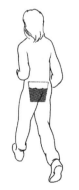

Figure 3.50

it should be a gentle lifting motion (up and in) of the lower abdominal and buttocks muscles to keep the front of the pelvic brim up, level, and stable. Don't allow much twisting between the various body "blocks"; that is, keep the front of your face, chest, and pelvis relatively stable and facing forward. Think of walking more quietly and smoothly by using the muscles of your feet and legs. As you continue walking, think about how stably and smoothly you are moving.

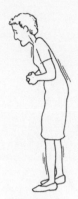

Figure 3.51

▼ Bad Move: Careful/Stiff/Uptight Walk (FIG. 3.51)

This tendency may originate from structural stiffness. It may also stem from your fear of falling or your fear of setting off your pain simply by walking. It makes you look stiff—as if you're wearing a corset from head to toe. You are moving like a child who is carrying a bowl full of water across the room and is anxious about spilling it. Your muscles are working too hard because you're trying to prevent motion from occurring around your neck and/or back, and this excessive muscle activity pulls the joints together. Pain can result from the joints being crunched together and/or the muscles overworking and tightening up. This pattern results in fatigue. It's like having your emergency brake on while you are attempting to move forward.

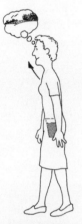

Figure 3.52

Excessive muscle guarding and/or tightness may tend to pull you in a particular direction. Common postures include the following: head down and forward, shoulders elevated, chest held down, abdomen clenched, and buttocks muscles tense.

▲ Good Move: Release Tension as You Walk (FIG. 3.52)

Take a few Cleansing and Calming Breaths. As you inhale, think of the air circulating to your areas of tension. Feel how the air allows these tense areas to relax and become lighter. As you exhale, think of releasing the tightness that is holding your body too rigidly together. Get rid of the bad air! Think of the water in your pelvic bowl—move such that the water becomes tranquil.

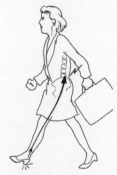

Figure 3.53

▼ Bad Move: Heel-Pounding Walk (FIG. 3.53)

This pattern of walking is characterized by a heavy heel/foot strike. It tends to send increased shock waves up the leg that can put stress on any of the pelvic or spinal joints. This kind of walking is probably a habit, and it's usually more exaggerated when you are in a hurry, angry, barefoot, or wearing flat shoes with dense, hard heels or spike high heels.

▲ Good Move: Impose a Smooth, Efficient Landing of Your Heel and Foot As You Walk (FIG. 3.54)

Think about landing quietly, smoothly, and efficiently. This will cause you to use more muscle control in your feet and legs, and a smoother carriage will result. Make sure that your shoes are not contributing to your pounding (for example, shoes with solid, dense heels or insoles that offer little shock absorption). Better shoes or a pair of cushion insoles will probably help. However, the most important thing is to make sure you reduce the degree of pounding by simply thinking about landing more smoothly, quietly, and softly. As you improve your ability to land softly, you can walk as swiftly as you wish.

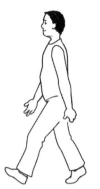

Figure 3.54

▼ Bad Move: Stress Walking (FIG. 3.55)

Stress walking typically includes fast, choppy walking with the head and trunk held relatively down and forward. Your facial expression (frowning, clenching the jaw, etc.) usually indicates that things are not going well. Muscle tension is usually significantly increased around your typical pain areas. This pattern of walking is akin to straining while on the toilet.

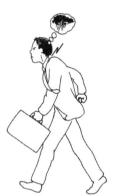

Figure 3.55

▲ Good Move: Mellow Walking (FIG. 3.56)

Try to imagine that everything is OK. Allow your stride to slow down and lengthen, letting momentum rather than tension carry you ahead. Allow the head and trunk to be relatively upright in order to improve your ventilation. Change your

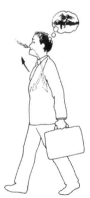

Figure 3.56

facial expression to what you want to be feeling (happy, confident, tranquil, etc.). Concentrate on moving symmetrically and in good alignment—release tension and "bad vibes" through easy movement, exhalation, and positive images.

Improving Your Footwear

The way your shoe responds to the ground and the way your foot responds to the shoe will be transmitted up your leg to various body "blocks"; therefore, the kind of shoe you wear can significantly affect how you feel while standing and walking. Regardless of the style of shoe you wear, you should consider the basic criteria described below. (Consult with your therapist about advisable heel height, as this varies from person to person.)

HEEL COUNTER (FIG. 3.57): This is like the keel of a boat; it needs to be stable enough to hold your heel upright while you stand and walk.

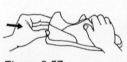

Figure 3.57

♦ *Desirable:* The heel counter should comfortably cup the back and sides of the heel and should be able to hold this area upright as you walk. The material used must be reinforced and sturdy enough to remain stable even after the shoes are no longer new.

♦ *Problematic:* A flimsy heel counter is one that can be collapsed if you press your finger on it. This allows the heel to move around too much, especially to tilt inward or outward. If your heel tilts outward, the ankle tends to be in a more rigid position so that more shock may be transmitted up the leg to the spine. If your heel falls inward, the foot arches tend to get flattened out. This may increase strain up the leg to the lower back.

HEEL: This is the platform under your heel bone.

◆ *Desirable:* The heel should be well padded for shock absorption and should be supported approximately ½–¾" higher than the ball of the foot. Also, the width of the heel should be equal to the width of the heel counter; this will help to "spread out" the strain forces and therefore improve shock absorption.

◆ *Problematic:* Hard, dense heels increase the amount of shock transmitted up the leg to the spine. Flat heels may increase shock due to the dense material used. Narrow, spiky heels cause a wobbling effect up the leg that may increase muscle tension in problem areas. Mushy, spongy heels may increase strain because they "give" too much and because they are usually combined with a flimsy heel counter. Heels that have become worn and uneven may aggravate your alignment and muscle tension. Don't let them go too far before you get them repaired or replaced.

FLEXIBILITY (Fig. 3.58):

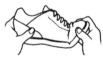

Figure 3.58

◆ *Desirable:* When you attempt to bend the shoe, it should "give" at the ball of the foot to provide smooth rollover. When the shoe is on, you should be able to scrunch, extend, and wiggle your toes.

◆ *Problematic:* If the shoe is too rigid, it will not "give" when you try to bend it; this certainly can be uncomfortable. Also, constantly wearing tight, inflexible shoes can "retard" a foot—the foot doesn't have a chance to respond to the ground because the shoe won't let it.

If the shoe is too flimsy, it will collapse at various areas along the sole, or it will twist, allowing problem foot positions.

If worn consistently, flimsy shoes allow your foot to "collapse" easier, perhaps leading to fallen arches.

INSOLE (FIG. 3.59): On the inside of the shoe, this is the material on the flat foot surface that goes from the heel to the toes.

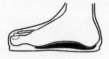

Figure 3.59

◆ *Desirable:* The insole should provide comfortable support to the heel and the arch on the inside of the foot. As you run your finger over this area on the inside of the shoe, you should feel a rise in the contour of the material that matches the height of your own arch. The cushioning should extend from the heel at least to the ball of the foot.

◆ *Problematic:* If there is no stable build-up of material in the arch area, it will be easy to push the material of the shoe over the side. This may occur as you walk, allowing the foot to flatten out. Combining flat, hard insoles with dense heels can add painful compression to the leg and spine.

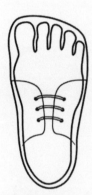

Figure 3.60

TOE BOX: This is the area that surrounds the toes from the bottom to the top on the inside of the shoe.

◆ *Desirable:* (FIG. 3.60): The toe box should allow adequate height and width so that the toes can be wiggled, scrunched, and raised slightly. The walls of the toe box should be close enough to the foot to keep the foot from sliding around.

◆ *Problematic:* (FIG. 3.61): Shoes that "bind" the foot and toes belong to another culture and time. Your toes should not be scrunched, pinched, or crammed. You should not feel the topside of your toes hitting the roof of the toe box.

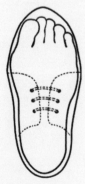

Figure 3.61

FOCUS ON BENDING AND LIFTING

On most days, you frequently bend over to pick up various objects and to complete numerous tasks. If you exhibit bad bending form, you put a significant amount of pressure and strain on your spine. Repeatedly or consistently exhibiting bad bending form can continue and increase your pain problem even if you're not picking up anything heavier than a shoe. On the other hand, use of good form while bending and lifting can promote the following benefits: increased leg and trunk strength; improved ability to bend and lift in comfort; decreased risk of re-injury or re-aggravation of your symptoms; and improved ability to lift heavier objects. Using good form while bending may be one of the most effective things you can do to reduce the rounding effect that gravity has on your spine over the years. Lifting correctly throughout the day creates "opportunistic exercise" in your daily activity. Using good squatting form while lifting exercises your bigger muscles so you are exercising as you lift.

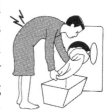

Figure 3.62a

▼ Bad Bending and Lifting Moves

▼ Feet too close together: If your feet are closer than shoulder width apart, you'll have poor leverage, will be unstable, and will tend to round out your back (FIG. 3.62a).

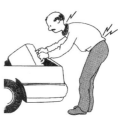

Figure 3.62b

▼ Knees and hips straight, with lower back rounded forward: This is the most common and stressful bad move during lifting, especially if done while twisting the trunk (FIG. 3.62b).

▼ Tensing and arching the neck up: This crams the neck joints together and becomes a pain, especially if maintained for awhile (as when gardening) or during heavy lifting (FIG. 3.62c).

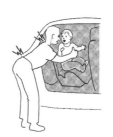

Figure 3.62c

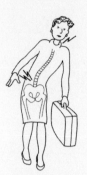

Figure 3.63

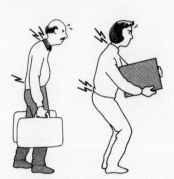

Figure 3.64

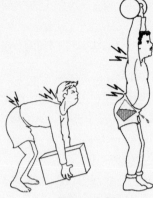

Figure 3.65

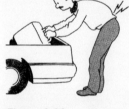

Figure 3.66

▼ Lifting and carrying an imbalanced load (FIG. 3.63).

▼ Lifting and bending too much in a short period of time: If you start getting tired, you'll start slumping, which causes increased compression and strain (FIG. 3.64).

▼ Lifting objects that are too heavy for you (FIG. 3.65): This will typically result in attempting to jerk-lift and/or to lift in a slumped or overarched posture. If you can't lift slowly and smoothly in good alignment, don't attempt it!

▼ Lifting heavy objects right after sustained sitting, especially if you've been slump sitting: This is a bad, dangerous combination! (FIG. 3.66)

▼ Overhead reaching or lifting, with the neck and lower back overarched (FIG. 3.67).

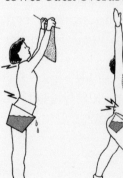

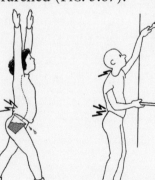

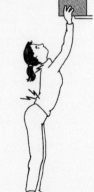

Figure 3.67

▲ Good Bending and Lifting Moves

▲ Place feet and knees at least shoulder width apart or front to back in a wide-step position. This helps you to bend at the hips, keeping the back relatively straight and unstressed (FIG. 3.68a, b, and d).

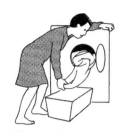

Figure 3.68a

▲ Lean over or squat with the chest and buttocks sticking out. If this move is done correctly, your back will be straight and the neck will balance in a relaxed, neutral position (FIG. 3.68a, d, and e).

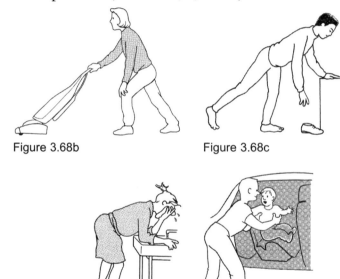

Figure 3.68b

Figure 3.68c

Figure 3.68d

Figure 3.68e

▲ Take weight through one or both arms. As you squat down or push back up, prop your hand or elbow on your thigh, the furniture, a wall, countertops, etc. This good move takes some of the compression and strain off the lower back (FIG. 3.68a, c, and d).

▲ When possible, balance your load on either side; or at least switch sides so that both sides are stressed fairly equally (FIG. 3.69).

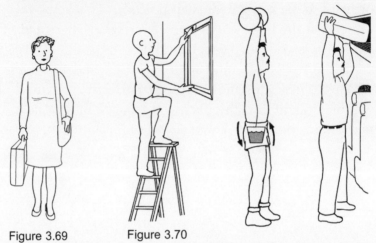

Figure 3.69   Figure 3.70

▲ When reaching or lifting overhead, level the pelvis (see p. 74), keep the chest up, and/or use a step stool to keep the lower back and neck in neutral alignment (FIG. 3.70).

▲ Prior to or after sustained bending or heavy lifting, walk around and use the Backward Bending and/or Stomach Lying positions, especially if you've been sitting awhile (see pp. 18 and 17).

Healthy Bending and Lifting Options

The following options are consistent with the good moves just presented and can be used for most bending and lifting functions:

UMPIRE SQUAT (FIG. 3.71a): Position your feet wider than shoulder width apart; bear weight on your thighs with your hands, forearms, or elbows. Keep your chest up and your back straight as you lower and rise, bending and straightening at the hips and knees.

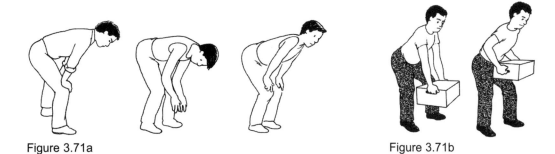

Figure 3.71a   Figure 3.71b

SQUAT LIFT (FIG. 3.71b): Maintain your chest up and your back straight as you push up with your legs. Your arms should "lock in"; that is, you should hold the weight of the object up and close to you, without allowing your chest to be slumped down as you lift. When lifting heavier objects from a full squat, keeping your elbows or forearms in contact with the insides of your legs helps make you more stable and transfers more weight off the spine and onto the legs.

SUPPORTED LEG LIFT BEND (FIG. 3.72): Slide or raise a leg out behind you as you bend at the hip of the standing leg. This helps you keep the spine relatively straight and unstressed. Take weight through your arm or arms as you bend at the hips. This technique is easier on the knees and does not require as much leg flexibility and strength as the Umpire Squat. If you have one-sided low back or leg pain, take the weight off the problematic leg as you bend over the opposite leg. This technique is only good for lifting lightweight objects (clothing, small toys, a newspaper, etc.) that can be handled easily with one hand. Rise up by straightening the standing leg and pushing up through your "prop" arm.

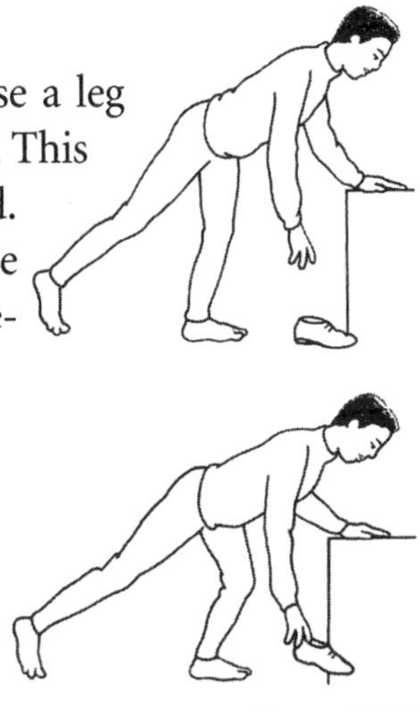

Figure 3.72

> **CAUTION: AVOID THIS TECHNIQUE IF YOU ARE PREGNANT, OR IF YOU SUSPECT OR HAVE BEEN TOLD THAT YOUR PELVIC JOINTS ARE LOOSE.**

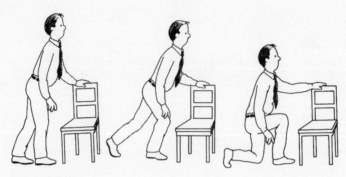

Figure 3.73

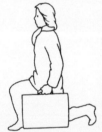

LUNGE TO HALF-KNEELING (FIG. 3.73): This technique is typically a bit easier than performing a full squat. It's also quite useful when you are feeling especially cautious about bending because you are experiencing increased pain. Once you are in the half-kneeling position, it's great for performing sustained light work that's low to the ground.

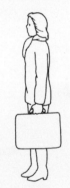

Figure 3.74

HALF-KNEELING LIFT (FIG. 3.74): This is a good technique for lifting groceries and suitcases. Once in the half-kneeling position, simply push up through both legs to standing. Keep your chest up tall (don't bend over) as you lift; keep the arms tense to keep the weight from pulling you down into a slumped position. For heavier boxes that are on the ground and without handles, use the half-kneeling position to roll the box onto your down thigh (FIG. 3.75). Once you have your arms under it and it is pulled close to your body, push up with your legs from half-kneeling to standing. Again, make sure to keep the back straight.

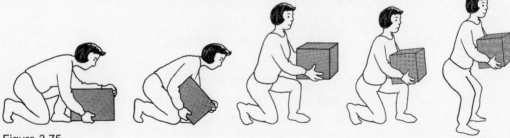

Figure 3.75

Good Moves/Bad Moves
During Daily Activities:
Key Concepts

let-go tests while sitting and standing: These tests involve producing your exaggerated poor alignment by essentially letting go and allowing yourself to view your worst alignment. These tests are not meant to be repeated as an exercise; use them only in the beginning, till you are aware of your exaggerated poor alignment; after that, perform your postural adjustment exercise by simply sitting or standing in your comfortable alignment and then proceeding directly to your exaggerated good alignment.

exaggerated good alignment: As you perform the postural adjustment exercises, your body will move from poor alignment to this alignment. Exaggerated good alignment represents almost an overcorrection of your postural alignment that you consciously hold and look at for short periods of time (10–30 seconds); this overcorrection will help to change your postural "computer" so that it learns that this improved alignment is you. This way, when you relax and let go of holding yourself in the exaggerated good alignment, your body will return to a more neutral improved alignment; that is, it will not return totally to your poor alignment for a while. Over time, by repeating the postural adjustment exercises that move you into exaggerated good alignment numerous times on a daily basis, you will actually change your posture toward this improved alignment.

neutral alignment: This refers to the optimal balance of the body "blocks" from front to back and side to side. You achieve neutral position by getting into exaggerated good alignment, then gradually relaxing; the resulting improved alignment is your neutral position for the time being; it can gradually improve over time. In general, your neutral position should be your most comfortable position.

CHAPTER 4

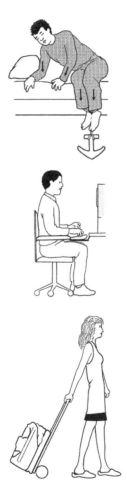

Wheel of Function

❦

A.M. RISING

BATHING AND DRESSING

COMMUTING

AT THE OFFICE OR
IN THE CLASSROOM

HOUSE AND YARD WORK

TRAVEL AND LEISURE

BEDTIME

This chapter tells you how to improve your comfort, productivity, and physical health while you perform such everyday tasks as getting out of bed, bathing, commuting, and doing office work or housework. For each of these tasks, you will be shown patterns to avoid (bad moves) and patterns to be encouraged (good moves). In reading this chapter, concentrate on those tasks and situations that you encounter on a daily basis, especially those that typically increase your pain.

A.M. RISING

Before Getting out of Bed

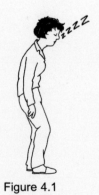

Figure 4.1

If your body feels especially stiff, tense, slumped, or heavy in the morning, it may be beneficial to perform a few simple movement/breathing exercises before you even get out of bed. This will serve to relubricate your joints, ventilate your lungs, and prepare your structure for all the movement that is needed in the morning. This process naturally takes place when you stretch and yawn. It's a good move to add a few extra moments of comfortable, healthy stretching and deep breathing before getting out of bed.

AVOID GETTING UP SLUMPED AND ROUNDED: If you sleep in a curled-up position, and/or feel rounded and stooped over when you first attempt to get up in the morning (FIG. 4.1), take a few moments to first lengthen out your body while you're still in bed. Instead of slumping through your morning, attempt any of the following good moves before or soon after getting up (FIG. 4.2).

- ◆ Back Lying Extension Rest Position (pp. 16–17)
- ◆ Stomach Lying (p. 17)
- ◆ Stomach Lying on Elbows (pp. 17–18)
- ◆ Pressups (pp. 148–149)
- ◆ Spinal Counter Rotation (pp. 142–145)

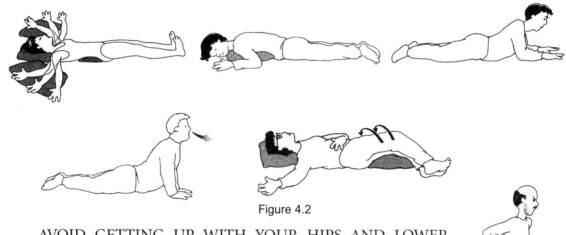

Figure 4.2

AVOID GETTING UP WITH YOUR HIPS AND LOWER BACK STIFF AND TIGHT (FIG. 4.3): If you tend to sleep flat-out on your stomach or back, or if you simply feel it's difficult to bend over or straighten up because of low back and hip tightness/stiffness, do a few moments of gentle loosening up to help yourself stand up straight and bend down with less stress/pain. Try any of the following good moves before or soon after getting up (FIG. 4.4):

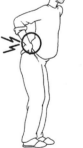

Figure 4.3

◆ Knees to Chest (pp. 146–148)
◆ Hands and Knees Rocking and Shifting (pp. 149–151)
◆ Hip Flexor Stretches (pp. 159–161)
◆ Lower Abdominal Isometric (pp. 164–165)

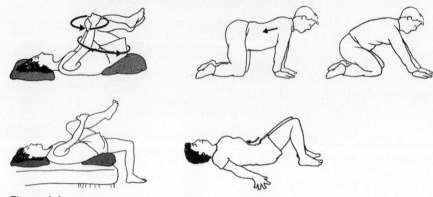

Figure 4.4

IF YOUR NECK OR SHOULDERS FEEL STIFF, TIGHT, OR TENSE WHEN YOU FIRST GET UP, TRY ANY OF THE FOLLOWING (FIG. 4.5):

◆ Neck Straightening and Decompression (pp. 27–29)
◆ Neck Release (pp. 29–30)
◆ Spinal Counter Rotation (pp. 142–145)

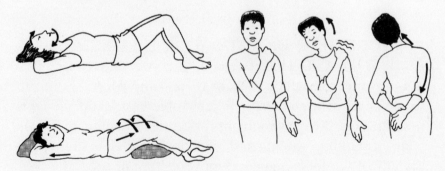

Figure 4.5

Sitting Up

AVOID "STRUGGLING" TO GET UP (Fig. 4.6): Don't attempt to pull your head and spine directly up against the forces of gravity. When getting up from any position, avoid tensing the front of the neck to pull forward; this simply strains the soft tissues in this area and squashes the joints together—ouch!

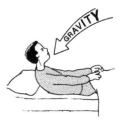

Figure 4.6

ATTEMPT TO USE GRAVITY AND MOMENTUM TO GET UP TO SITTING. TRY LOG ROLLING (Fig. 4.7): This involves rolling the head, neck, trunk, pelvis, and legs simultaneously so that little twisting occurs among these areas. Keep your breathing and the muscles along your spine relatively relaxed; that is, don't tighten up your neck or abdomen. Instead, allow the synchronized rolling weight of your body and gravity to do the work. The weight of your legs is the "anchor weight"; allow their lowering toward the ground to pull you up as you simultaneously push up with your arms. As you lower your legs, keep facing the bed where your arms are pushing—otherwise gravity will tend to pull you onto your backside. This method can be done slowly if you're feeling cautious and uncomfortable, or it can be done very quickly if you're feeling well. Either way, this good move reduces much of the force on the spine and is a more efficient way of getting up to a sitting position.

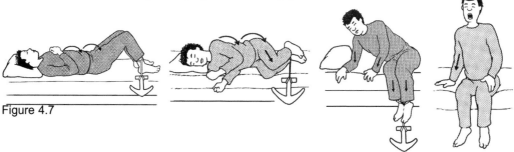

Figure 4.7

Standing Up

This involves changing from the sitting "gear" to the standing "gear." First thing in the morning, the spine and pelvis often have difficulty changing gears. After you've been relatively immobile all night, it can be an uncomfortable shock to attempt "popping up" into the standing gear.

▼ BAD MOVES (FIG. 4.8):

 ▼ Avoid sitting slumped on the side of the bed, especially if you're on a soft mattress where you'll tend to sink in.

 ▼ As you stand up, avoid bending over. Try not to "round" the lower back and drop the head forward before you attempt to straighten up. (Keep in mind that if you're looking down at the ground, you'll tend to bend over excessively.)

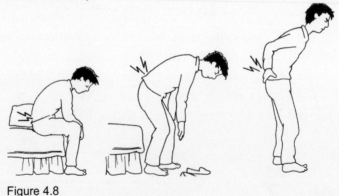

Figure 4.8

▲ GOOD MOVES:

 ▲ Attempt to sit tall and gently arch the lower back up and forward before standing. (FIG. 4.9a).

 ▲ Bend forward at the hips, keeping your back straight (FIG. 4.9b).

▲ Bring one foot slightly behind the other; keep your pelvis level as you simultaneously straighten your legs and shift from your back foot to your front foot (FIG. 4.9c).

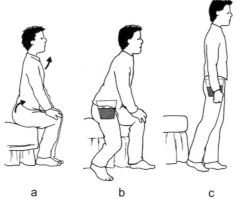

Figure 4.9   a   b   c

Note: If you're having difficulty standing up because your bed is too low and/or soft, try putting a bed board in or getting a new mattress to help firm up your "launching pad."

BATHING AND DRESSING

On the Toilet

▼ BAD MOVES (FIG. 4.10):

▼ Avoid slumping, straining, and holding your breath. Pushing hard through the rectum while slumping is an especially aggravating move for the lower back.

▼ Avoid clenching your jaw and tensing the neck and facial muscles. These are common habits that add painful stress to the neck region.

▼ Avoid holding your breath. This causes increased stress throughout your system.

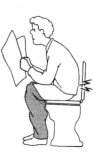

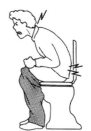

Figure 4.10

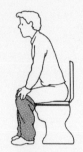

▲ GOOD MOVES (FIG. 4.11a):

    ▲ Stay relaxed and up by repositioning your pelvis (see pp. 52–53) and using your arms to help support you.

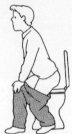

    ▲ Take a few Cleansing Breaths or simply maintain relaxed breathing—release any tense holding of muscles as you exhale.

    ▲ Stand up by pushing through your arms and legs, keeping your trunk up and tall—that is, no bending over prior to standing.

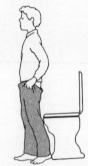

    ▲ During periods of acute low back pain, use of a raised toilet seat will help if you find it painful to sit on the toilet or to go from sitting to standing (FIG. 4.11b).

At the Sink

▼ BAD MOVES (FIG. 4.12):

    ▼ Avoid bad bending form, especially slumping or arching forward with the legs straight, without support.

    ▼ Avoid sticking your neck and chin out to an unnecessary degree as you stand in front of the mirror to shave, apply makeup, or brush your teeth.

Figure 4.11a

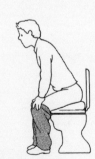

Figure 4.11b

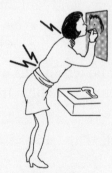
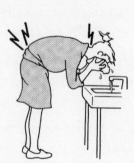

Figure 4.12

▼ Avoid tensing and arching your neck up as you bend over the sink to rinse.

▲ GOOD MOVES:

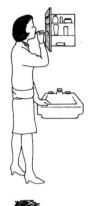

▲ When shaving, applying makeup, or brushing your teeth, take weight through at least one arm; place one foot up; level your pelvis by holding in your buttocks and lower abdominal muscles (see pp. 70–72) or placing a step under or alongside the sink; use an adjustable mirror or change your position (sit or stand on the side of the sink with the mirror open toward you—this way you don't have to stick your neck out or lean as far over the sink) (FIG. 4.13).

▲ When bending over to rinse, move your feet wider than shoulder width apart; attempt taking weight through at least one arm; squat or use the Supported Leg Lift Bend (see p. 89) (that is, raise and lower yourself by bending at your hips, not your back, and keep the back straight) (FIG. 4.14).

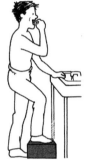

Figure 4.13

▲ When sneezing, coughing, clearing your throat, or blowing your nose, avoid forceful bending, "whiplash" movements and tension that stress the head, neck, and lower back (FIG. 4.15).

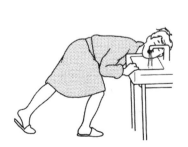

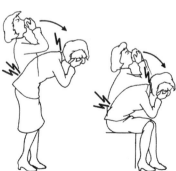

Figure 4.14

Figure 4.15

Instead, attempt to stabilize yourself in an upward position with an arm on the sink or wall. When blowing your nose, lean back against the wall to keep from bending forward. Let the force of the cough or sneeze go through your extended arm, instead of your neck and lower back (FIG. 4.16).

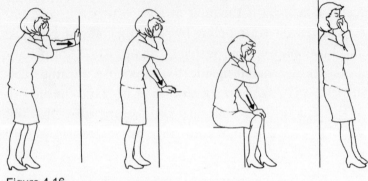

Figure 4.16

In the Shower

▼ BAD MOVES (FIG. 4.17):

    ▼ Avoid staying bent over while you wash and dry your front, shave your legs, etc.

    ▼ Avoid slumping over to adjust the faucets, pick up the soap, or wash/dry your legs without taking weight through your arms.

    ▼ Avoid rolling your head backward to intentionally crack your neck.

▲ GOOD MOVES (FIG. 4.18):

    ▲ Attempt to maintain your head, trunk, and pelvis in a relaxed, upright alignment while you wash and dry; reach with your arms instead of twisting and bending your trunk; squat to lower your head under the spray.

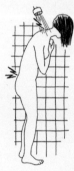

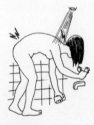

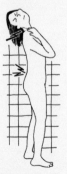

Figure 4.17

▲ When washing and drying your legs and feet, prop one foot up onto the tub rim or a bath stool; take weight through your arms and squat, using the other leg to lower yourself. Keep your chest up and your neck relaxed.

▲ Shower massagers and self-massage with the soothing heat of the shower can reduce muscle tension and stiffness. Release and lengthening exercises often work well when performed in the shower.

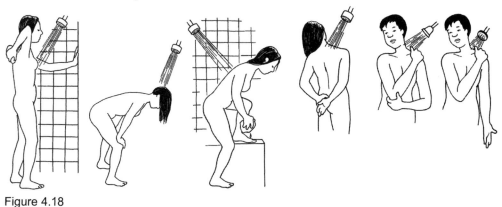

Figure 4.18

In the Tub

▼ BAD MOVES (FIG. 4.19):

▼ Avoid long periods of lying with the spine in a rounded, curled position, or with the neck arched excessively backward on the tub rim.

▼ Avoid bending over to wash your feet with your legs straight and your back rounded.

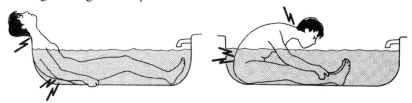

Figure 4.19

▲ GOOD MOVES (FIG. 4.20):

▲ Support yourself in more relaxed, upright alignments. Neck and low back supports for the tub are commercially available, or you can simply use rolled towels
to put behind your lower back and neck/head. Reposition your pelvis first (see pp. 52–53), and then place the
towel behind you.

▲ When washing your legs and feet, bring them up to
you one at a time, while staying relaxed and supported
through the trunk.

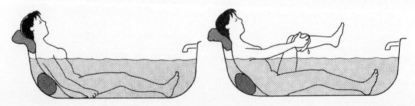

Figure 4.20

While Dressing

▼ BAD MOVES (FIG. 4.21):

▼ Avoid unsupported slumping when picking up
shoes and reaching into low drawers.

▼ Avoid unsupported and/or slumped alignment
while dressing your lower limbs.

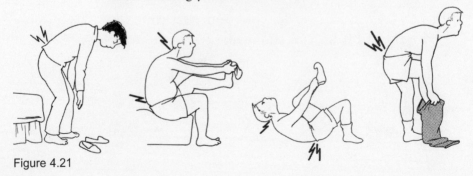

Figure 4.21

▲ GOOD MOVES:

▼ If you wish to dress while sitting, sit in a chair with a firm seat; if you sit on the edge of the bed, raise it and firm it up by sitting on a pillow. To put on your shoes and socks, keep your back straight, bring your foot up to you, and cross your legs or place your heel on the edge of the seat (FIG. 4.22a).

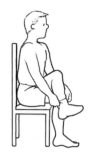

Figure 4.22a

▼ If you wish to bend over, bend at the hips (not the spine) so the lower back stays relatively straight, and take weight through an arm (FIG. 4.22b).

▼ When dressing while standing, prop back against a counter or wall to avoid some of the compression and strain of bending over. Attempt to bend your legs up to step into pants or a skirt (instead of bending the spine over and down) (FIG. 4.22c).

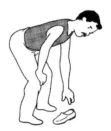

Figure 4.22b

▼ If you put your shoes and socks on while standing, bring your foot up onto a chair bench or the bed (FIG. 4.22d).

▼ During more acute episodes, bending over to dress may really aggravate your low back pain; if this is the case, try partially dressing your lower limbs while lying on your back (FIG. 4.22e).

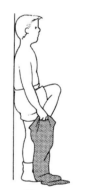

Figure 4.22c

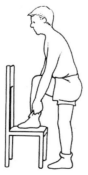

Figure 4.22d

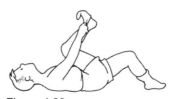

Figure 4.22e

COMMUTING

Commuting largely involves sitting, so review the "Focus on Sitting" section of chapter 3. Additional recommendations specific to commuting include the following:

ATTEMPT RELAXED, UPRIGHT COMMUTING: Your most important move should be done right away and should be repeated throughout your commute: this move is Pelvic Repositioning (see pp. 52–53), which can be used in the Back and Up and Forward and Up positions.

The Back and Up position (see p. 55) allows you to relax back in a slightly reclined position. Move your seat up so you can easily reach the pedals, and recline the backrest 5–15 degrees. Occasionally push your arms straight on the steering wheel (if driving) or onto your thighs (if a passenger); this will help to decompress your lower back and pelvis. Periodically arch your lower back forward away from the backrest (FIG. 4.23).

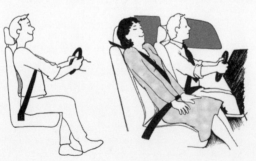

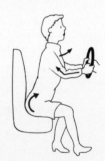

Figure 4.23   Figure 4.24

Use the Forward and Up position (see p. 55) when you feel as though you need to decrease the pressure against your back. It's also helpful when you're in busy traffic, or when visibility is a problem. For extra decompression and relaxation to the lower back, you can gently pull up on the steering wheel to lift weight up off the spine (save this for when you are stopped at intersections) (FIG. 4.24).

(These good moves can also be performed on planes, trains, and buses.)

IF YOU FEEL LIKE YOU ARE TENSING UP and/or experiencing increased pain because of a bumpy or swervy ride, reposition your pelvis into the Forward and Up position and use your arms as shock absorbers by placing your hands on your thighs or on the seat beside you; this will decrease the strain forces going through the spine. Allow your body to sway slowly and gently with the bumpy or swervy motion (like a giant Jell-O mold)—don't attempt to hold yourself stiffly, as this will only result in more shock and irritation.

IF YOU ARE DRIVING OR RIDING IN YOUR OWN CAR, OR IF YOU ARE FLYING OR RIDING ON A BUS OR TRAIN, ASSESS THE NEED FOR IMPROVED SUPPORT. For example, if you slump when you relax and let go, you may benefit by leveling the seat (p. 58), using a lumbar support (pp. 59–61), and/or taking weight off your spine by using an armrest. Keep your supports in the car or take them with you on the plane, train, or bus so you'll use them.

AVOID KEEPING YOUR HEAD TURNED TO ONE SIDE TOO LONG. This tends to cram the neck joints together and tense up the muscles on the side toward which you're looking. If this happens, sit up tall with your chin in and slowly turn your head to the opposite side for a few seconds and take a deep Cleansing Breath. This will usually "straighten you out" and give some immediate relief.

WHEN TRAFFIC PERMITS, USE ONE HAND TO PROVIDE SELF-MASSAGE to tight, sensitive areas around the neck and tops of the shoulders (FIG. 4.25; see pp. 40–42). When at stops, move the head around and take a few Cleansing Breaths to release any tense holding.

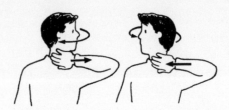

Figure 4.25

AVOID POOR ALIGNMENT WHILE NAPPING AND/OR READING ON THE BUS, PLANE, OR TRAIN. Reposition yourself and use a support (briefcase, packages, etc.) to relax yourself in good alignments.

STAND, STRETCH, AND WALK TALL FROM YOUR TRANSPORTATION TO YOUR JOB. With a little awareness and effort, you can turn this everyday event into an effective part of your exercise regime. Lengthen, strengthen, and reventilate your body before arriving at the workplace by getting off the bus or out of the car a few blocks earlier and walking. Wear supportive and comfortable shoes. Stay relaxed and attempt to use good walking form (see the "Focus on Walking" section of chapter 3).

At the Office or in the Classroom

The office and classroom environments primarily involve sustained sitting and, often, a good deal of stress. So to keep your body balanced, (1) use a variety of good sitting alternatives; (2) stand, walk, and stretch between work functions; and (3) occasionally take a few Cleansing Breaths and mental vacations. These methods should be reviewed in the "Focus on Sitting" section of chapter 3. Additional recommendations will be made here; focus on the ones that seem to apply to you.

Reading, Writing, Typing, Xeroxing, etc.

AVOID THE SUSTAINED HEAD-DOWN POSITION (FIG. 4.26): Regardless of whether you are slumping or sitting up tall, doing these eye-hand activities on a flat surface that is too low or with your materials too close to the edge will require you to look down at an angle that will pull your head and neck down and forward.

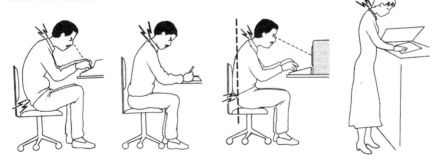

Figure 4.26

REPOSITION YOURSELF: While sitting, the first step to getting your head back into a balanced position is to reposition your pelvis (see pp. 52–53). Also, when reading, try sitting with your chair positioned sideways to your desk. This way you can rest one arm on the desk, which decreases the forward bending forces on the spine.

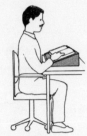

Figure 4.27a

CONSIDER USING A SLANT BOARD TO SAVE YOUR NECK (FIG. 4.27a): By simply elevating and slanting your writing or reading surface and/or typewriter, you will decrease the bend between the head and neck. By allowing a more "level-headed" position, slant boards can significantly reduce strain to muscular and joint tissues. Try placing your materials on a large three-ring binder; even this slight change in angle is usually enough to make you notice a positive difference. Slant boards can usually be found in art and drafting supply stores, self-help catalogues, or through occupational therapy departments.

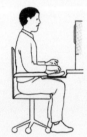

Figure 4.27b

CONSIDER USING ARMRESTS AT THE PROPER HEIGHT (FIG. 4.27b): Placing armrests at the proper height will not only support the arms but also take pressure off the neck and shoulders. To determine the proper armrest height, sit in a comfortable, relaxed, and upright position. The armrests should be high enough and close enough to the body to support your arms in this position. If the armrests are too high, your shoulders will shrug; if they are too low, you will have to slouch in order for your arms to meet them.

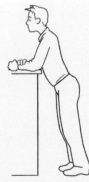

Figure 4.27c

IF YOU'VE BEEN SITTING TOO LONG ALREADY, SEEK OUT A TALL (CHEST/SHOULDER HEIGHT) FILE CABINET OR COUNTER that allows you to prop yourself up through your arms in order to read or write comfortably for a few minutes while standing (FIG. 4.27c).

CONSIDER USING FOOT RESTS: If by sitting back in your office chair you find that your feet don't touch the floor, you definitely need a foot rest—or, better yet, a chair with an adjustable height. If your feet are dangling, the muscles along the spine get activated, and neck or back pain is a common result. The foot rest should be high enough to support the feet without raising the knees up much higher than the hips. If it's the right height, you'll feel more comfortable right away. Note: If your chair back is not firm enough, using a foot rest may encourage slumping; in this case reposition your pelvis and get a lumbar support in there (see pp. 52–53).

SUPPORT YOUR HEAD TO RELAX YOUR NECK (FIG. 4.28): If you prop your head on your hand, the muscles around the neck can let go, and this unloads the joints. This is helpful during sustained writing or reading activities.

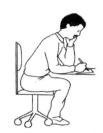

Figure 4.28

AVOID SUSTAINED USE OF COMPUTER SCREENS THAT PULL YOUR NECK OUT OF ALIGNMENT (FIG. 4.29): If a screen is too low, it will tend to pull your head and trunk down and forward (most common problem). If it is too high, it will tend to pull your head forward and arch it backward at the top. If it is too far off to one side, it can cause cramming of the joints and muscle tightness on the side toward which you've turned. If you combine any of these problematic positions with a screen that is too far away for easy visibility, you increase the probability of head, neck, shoulder, and/or low back pain even more.

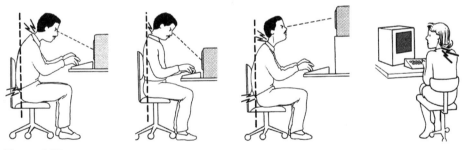

Figure 4.29

ATTEMPT REPOSITIONING YOUR COMPUTER SCREEN (FIG. 4.30): First of all, reposition your pelvis (see pp. 52–53) and support yourself into a comfortable, relaxed, upright position. Then position your monitor so that you do not have to tilt, turn, or move your head out of this alignment. If it is too low, elevate it to eye level so you can sit up tall and relaxed; if it's too high, bring it down so your chin is not sticking out. It should be either straight ahead or not more than a few degrees off to the side. If you prefer it slightly off to one side, try putting it on the side opposite the side on which you usually hold the phone. Make sure the screen is close enough so that you don't have to stick/drop your head forward to read it. A copy holder placed close to the monitor can reduce eye movements and prevent unnecessary turning of the head and neck.

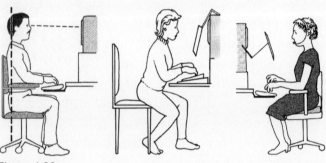

Figure 4.30

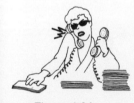

Figure 4.31

AVOID "WRINGING" YOUR NECK TO HOLD THE PHONE (FIG. 4.31): Holding the phone by scrunching your neck and shoulders together is commonly done to free up your hands. When you do this consistently over a period of time, it commonly aggravates or causes numerous pain problems in the head/neck and/or shoulders.

Attempt any of the following phone alternatives (FIG. 4.32):

◆ Hold the receiver in the hand opposite your writing hand; become aware enough to keep the shoulder and neck on this side relaxed (don't attempt to hold the phone with your shoulder or neck).

◆ Use commercially available phone rests that fit

onto the handle. These low-cost items help to stabilize the receiver onto your shoulder so that it will stay next to your ear and mouth without your tightening up to hold it there.

◆ Speaker phones and headsets are helpful devices to free up your hands and avoid stress on your neck and shoulder muscles.

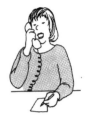

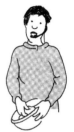

Figure 4.32

AVOID BENDING AND HANGING OVER FILES, DESKS, OR COUNTERS (FIG. 4.33): When pulling or replacing files in the lower file drawer, avoid bending over and staying bent over at the waist without propping through at least one of your arms.

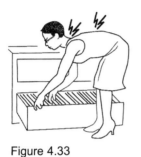

Figure 4.33   Figure 4.34

ATTEMPT GOOD BENDING FORM (FIG. 4.34): When bending over your desk top or when reaching into low drawers, take weight through one of your arms to avoid strain through the lower back. If you have to remain over a low file for more than a few seconds, kneel or prop weight through an arm.

Stretching at Your Desk

These exercises are meant to do the following: bring your spine and body parts into better alignment; ventilate your system; and release any build-up of excess muscle tension. Try them and do the ones that feel good to you!

PELVIC ROCKING AND HEAD/CHEST FLOATS (FIG. 4.35a

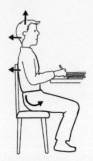

Figure 4.35a

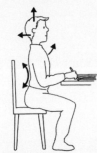

Figure 4.35b

and b): This is useful to do about once for every hour of sitting. It is especially good to do before getting up (see pp. 61–62).

SITTING LAID BACK AND UP (FIG. 4.36): Reposition your pelvis (see pp. 52–53) on the front part of the seat; lean back over the backrest, allowing your lower back to arch forward while you stretch your arms over your head; tuck your chin in gently, but allow your head to recline back with the trunk (you'll be looking up toward the ceiling in front of you, but not arching your neck backward); do a few Cleansing Breaths while lengthening your body.

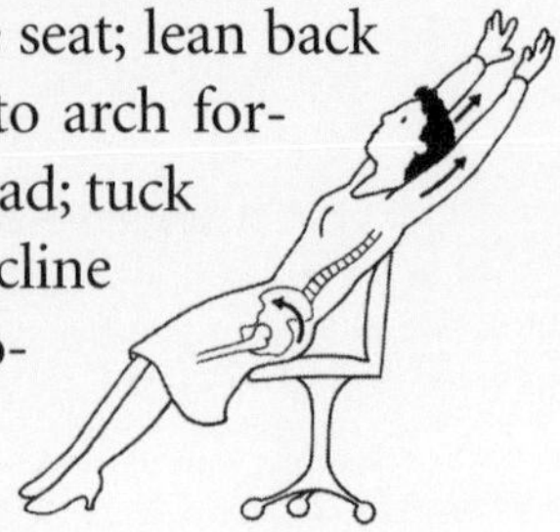

Figure 4.36

FORWARD SPINE RELEASE WHILE SITTING (FIG. 4.37): This is useful if your neck and/or back becomes uncomfortable because of sustained muscle tension, perhaps due to holding yourself still too long while working at your desk (uptight sitting).

Sit up tall in a relaxed, upright alignment with your arms propped on your thighs to take the weight off your spine. Take in a Cleansing Breath. As you exhale, allow your head to gradually release forward. As you allow your head to release forward, think of the vertebrae of your spine as links of a chain, and allow each "link" to release sequentially, from top to bottom. Stop lowering your body when you are naturally ready to inhale, or when the stretching sensation feels strong but productive. Then allow your body to slightly buoy up a bit as you inhale and to release a bit further down than before as you exhale. Continue this breathing and releasing pattern as you lower yourself further and further, releasing the lower neck, middle back, and lower back; take enough weight through your arms so you can release the tightness in a way that feels good and easy.

Use your arms to push yourself back upright to the starting position.

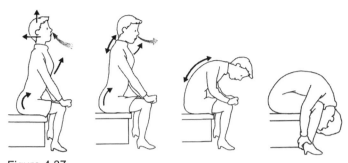

Figure 4.37

Note: You can release any separate portion of the spine (i.e., neck, middle back, lower back) without doing the whole exercise.

CAUTION: IF YOU FEEL THAT THIS EXERCISE TENDS TO INCREASE YOUR ARM, BUTTOCKS, OR LEG PAIN, DO NOT REPEAT IT. REPORT THESE SYMPTOMS TO YOUR DOCTOR OR PHYSICAL THERAPIST.

DESK TOP RESTING (FIG. 4.38): Roll your chair back away from your desk; reposition your pelvis; prop your arms on the desk and let your head rest on your forearms; allow your back to elongate and sag into a comfortable, forward-arched position; take a few Calming Breaths.

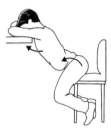

Figure 4.38

ROTATIONAL SPINE RELEASE WHILE SITTING (FIG. 4.39): After stretching tall while sitting, bring one arm to the outside of the opposite knee and turn so that you can reach and rest the other arm over the back of the chair. Gently turn your head, shoulders, and spine as far as you can in this same direction (keeping your knees straight ahead) till you feel a gentle, comfortable stretch. Pause there and take in a Cleansing Breath. As you exhale, allow your arms to twist your spine a little further if

your range opens up. Repeat this breathing/movement sequence 1–3 times before unwinding slowly and repeating it in
the opposite direction.

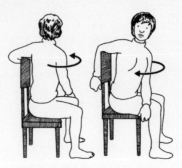

Figure 4.39

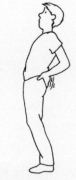

Figure 4.40

STANDING BACKWARD BENDING (FIG. 4.40): This is useful
when you have been sitting for an hour or more. Getting up and
gently reversing the direction of your spine is an effective way
to prevent tightness in the hips that can accumulate with sitting
too long. Standing backward bending will prepare your spine
and hips for standing and walking activities.

NECK RELEASE, NECK STRAIGHTENING AND DECOM-
PRESSION, AND SELF-MASSAGE (FIG. 4.41): During and/or
following activities that require you to hold your head still (typing, reading, etc.), it will be helpful to perform a few moments
of gentle straightening and lengthening combined with Cleansing and Calming Breaths.

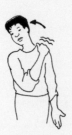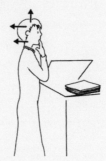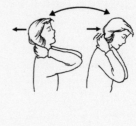

Figure 4.41

HOUSE AND YARD WORK

These tasks primarily involve bending, lifting, and repetitive movements. With a little awareness, and some improvements in your posture, these activities can become efficient and valuable forms of exercise. Refer back to the "Focus on Bending and Lifting" section of chapter 3 to review some of the good and bad moves associated with these universal tasks.

Housework

Vacuuming

Avoid the Neanderthal Method (FIG. 4.42): Oftentimes vacuuming will elicit your worst slumped or overarched alignment. Become aware of and decrease these bad moves by attempting these alternatives:

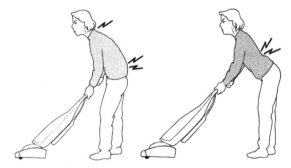

Figure 4.42

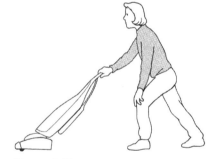

Figure 4.43

THE LUNGE (FIG. 4.43): Adopt a step position and posture as in the sport of fencing, with one leg stepping out in front. This way you can easily shift forward and back in various directions. As you step forward, you can reach forward with your vacuuming hand. Keep your pelvic "bowl" level. Put your other hand on your hip or thigh to take weight off the lower back and help you stay up. Attempt to change vacuuming hands every once in awhile.

KNEELING AND HALF-KNEELING (FIG. 4.44): These methods lower your center of gravity and automatically take some of the bend out of the activity. Try them as alternative positions for a few minutes. They're really comfortable!

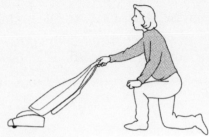

Figure 4.44

Dusting and Polishing (FIG. 4.45)

Prop your inactive arm on yourself or on the furniture to take more weight through your arms and less through your spine.

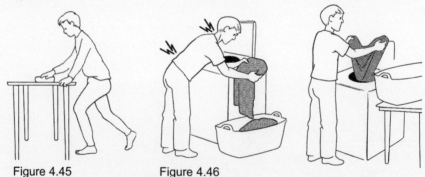

Figure 4.45   Figure 4.46

Doing the Laundry (FIG. 4.46)

Avoid slumped or overarched alignment when lifting, loading, and carrying. Load with one hand while taking weight through the other. Use exaggerated good alignment when lifting and carrying. Placing the laundry basket on a table or chair can decrease the amount of bending and lifting. Avoid overloading the basket.

Doing the Dishes, Ironing, Cleaning Windows (FIG. 4.47)

These tasks are similar to each other in that they involve sustained standing in a slightly forward-bent position. Place one foot up on a box or chair or inside the cabinet under the sink to help level your pelvic bowl and/or tense the muscles of your buttocks and lower abdomen to maintain your pelvis stable, level, and firmly up against the counter. For one-handed tasks, prop through your "resting" arm to take weight off the spine.

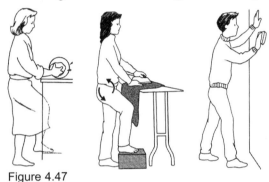

Figure 4.47

Making the Bed

AVOID SLUMPING OR ARCHING OUT OVER THE BED (FIG. 4.48). Lean up against the bed and bear weight through one arm when reaching.

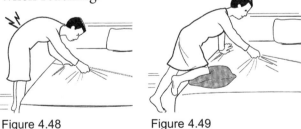

Figure 4.48   Figure 4.49

TRY SMOOTHING OUT THE SHEET AND TUCKING THE CORNERS WHILE KNEELING ON A PILLOW (FIG. 4.49). This makes the job much easier!

Yard Work

Mowing the Lawn (FIG. 4.50)

This can be a great strengthener. Maintain good alignment and relaxed breathing. Avoid slumping or overarching the lower back—keep your pelvis level (see p. 71–72). If the vibration of the mower seems to aggravate your symptoms, try thick gloves or use foam tape to insulate the handles.

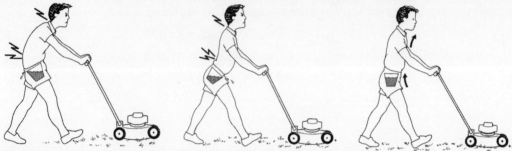

Figure 4.50

Gardening Low to the Ground (planting, weeding, edging) (FIG. 4.51)

Maintain good squatting methods. Refer to pages 88–89 for review. Also try kneeling, half-kneeling, and sitting on your heels. A number of helpful garden products assist with these positions, providing knee cushioning and something to push up off when getting up or down (an old pillow and a stake will assist in somewhat the same way). Be sure to stand, stretch up and backward, and walk after being in these bent-over positions.

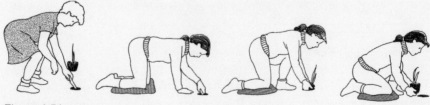

Figure 4.51

Sweeping/Raking (FIG. 4.52)

These activities are great overall strengtheners. Use an exaggerated, wide-base stance (feet wide apart) and keep your head, shoulders, pelvis, and feet balanced on top of each other and facing in the same direction (this insures minimal to no twisting). Reach and pull with your legs and arms, not your back. Rake and sweep in different directions by pivoting on your back leg and moving your whole body as a single, relaxed unit. Avoid looking down too close in toward your feet—rake/sweep about 1–2 feet in front of your feet. After sweeping or raking, do Neck Straightening and Decompression and Neck Release exercises (see pp. 27–31) for awhile if your neck feels stiff. Specially designed rakes with a bend in the stem do decrease the amount of necessary bending, so consider using them.

Reaching Up to Paint, Prune, Clean Windows (FIG. 4.53)

This can be a good upper back, arm, and abdominal strengthener. Use a ladder or step stool to keep from arching your lower back and letting your abdomen and buttocks stick out; make sure you keep your chest up, your pelvis level, and your head and neck in a neutral position. If you are uncomfortable after doing these activities, try doing the Knees to Chest, Neck Straightening and Decompression, and/or Neck Release exercises (see pp. 146–148 and 27–31).

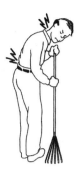

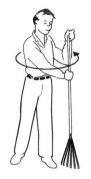

Figure 4.52

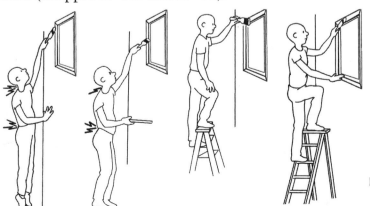

Figure 4.53

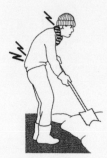

Figure 4.54a

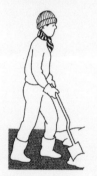

Figure 4.54b

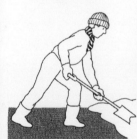

Figure 4.54c

Digging Holes/Shoveling Snow (FIG. 4.54)

CAUTION: These activities carry a high risk for aggravation and/or reinjury of most neck and low back problems; they are not good forms of exercise. If you have to perform these activities, avoid rounding out your spine while lifting (FIG. 4.54a). Keep the load light and manageable to avoid strain. Put your legs in a front-to-back step position and shift your weight through your legs. Keep your chest up and your buttocks sticking out—that is, squat instead of bend (FIG. 4.54 b and c). Keep your arms flexed and lift by straightening your legs. When you start to get tired or sore, stop! Stretch up and backward, walk, and wait awhile before deciding whether you should continue (if your pain does not totally disappear within a few minutes, pay the neighbor's kids to finish the job). Specially designed, bent-handled snow shovels (shown in FIG. 4.54b) make the job a little easier.

Washing the Car (FIG. 4.55)

This is a good strengthener for the arms and legs if you attempt good bending methods. Especially helpful are the Supported Leg Lift Method (see p. 89), squatting, and taking weight through both hands. Keep the lower back relatively straight and relaxed, and work those legs by squatting and shifting.

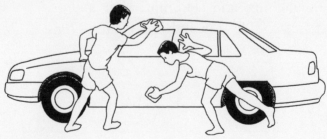

Figure 4.55

TRAVEL AND LEISURE

Travel

Packing

◆ Pack your suitcase on the bed or bureau—not on the floor! Put a foot up on the bed while folding and packing.

◆ Pack a balanced, light load.

◆ Take along "relief blankets"—cold packs, heating pads, low-level, continuous heat wraps—if any of these seem to help you.

Lifting/Carrying Luggage

Treat this as though it's a weightlifting workout—that is, avoid the bad moves shown in Figure 4.56 and attempt to use exaggerated good posture and good bending, lifting, and carrying methods.

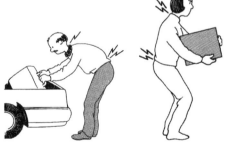

Figure 4.56

Here are some additional good moves:

◆ Be sure to carry a balanced, light load.

◆ Use portable luggage (FIG. 4.57). Make sure the handle is long enough that you don't have to bend and twist sideways while pulling, and make sure the rack can hold your luggage easily and securely. Full-size luggage carts are available for rent at most airports.

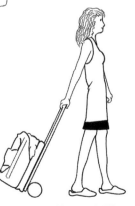
Figure 4.57

◆ Do not attempt to unload your luggage from the trunk or carry it until you've walked around a bit.

◆ If your pain is easily aggravated, see if you can get/pay someone to assist you.

◆ Avoid uptight walking (see p. 80), which can be caused by the weight of your bags as well as travel stress. Use Cleansing Breaths to help you release excess muscle tension.

◆ If you strain your back or neck/shoulder area by lifting or carrying your luggage, you should probably stretch out in a relief position and use ice as soon as you can.

◆ Wear good walking shoes. High heels, flats, or stiff, flimsy, or mushy shoes are no match for the athletic rigors of carrying, walking, and dodging in today's terminals!

Loading/Unloading the Car (FIG. 4.58)
This is a high-risk activity, so use caution.

◆ Put one foot on the bumper or in the trunk; that way, as you lift you simply transfer your weight from your front foot to your back foot. Prop through your other arm to assist with decompressing the spine.

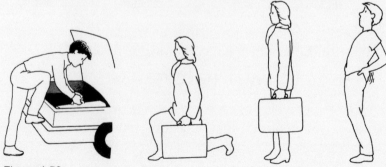

Figure 4.58

◆ Keep your back relatively straight (don't let it round out). Squat or move toward half-kneeling to pick up/lower the bags.

◆ Stretch up and back after setting the luggage down; and if you are tired or have any pain, stretch out on your stomach or back in a comfortable, decompressed position.

Sitting

Traveling usually means lots of sitting, so review the "Focus on Sitting" section of chapter 3.

◆ Move among the healthy sitting alternatives already recommended (see pp. 52–63).

◆ Bring along, or ask for, pillows to use under you, behind you, and as neck supports. If pillows are unavailable, improvise with clothing, magazines, etc.

◆ Occasionally take weight off the lower back by performing the following exercises: Sitting Laid Back and Up (FIG. 4.59a), Sitting Back and Up (FIG. 4.59b), and Sitting Forward and Up (FIG. 4.59c) (see pp. 54–55). Every hour, make sure you stop, stand, stretch, and walk.

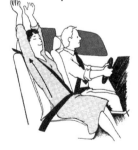
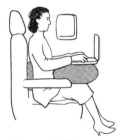
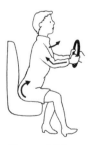

Figure 4.59a   Figure 4.59b   Figure 4.59c

◆ On long flights or train/bus rides, get up and walk to the farthest bathroom; if it's not choppy and there's room, stand for awhile and let yourself stretch and take a few Cleansing Breaths.

Leisure Time

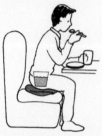

Leisure time generally involves sitting: at a restaurant or theater, at a card table, in a chair in front of the television, and so forth. Be sure to practice the sitting positions described in chapter 3, and keep in mind the following considerations.

◆ Most restaurant and theater seats do not offer adequate support in the right areas, so you may tend to slump or get uptight. The best solutions are to reposition your pelvis (see pp. 52–53); use a number of healthy sitting alternatives; use your coat, briefcase, purse, etc., under or behind you for extra support; and/or sit where it's convenient for you to get up without disturbing others (FIG. 4.60).

Figure 4.60

◆ Leisure positions can be harmful instead of restful. Avoid unsupportive "cushy" furniture that causes you to slump. Also avoid hard, unyielding surfaces that tend to strain you. Occasionally reposition your pelvis (see pp. 52–53) and consider using seat and lumbar supports to keep your body in line and comfortable (FIG. 4.61).

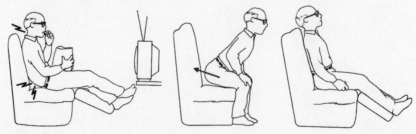

Figure 4.61

◆ If you're reading, writing, or sewing while sitting on a recliner, be sure to reposition your pelvis (see pp.

52–53) and use one or two large pillows in your lap to support your arms and to raise up what you're looking at (FIG. 4.62).

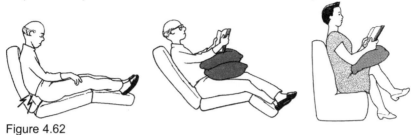

Figure 4.62

◆ As an alternative to always sitting, use your leisure time to do stretching and lengthening exercises; use relief positions and relief blankets; perform self-massage; lie down on the floor and exercise during television commercials (FIG. 4.63).

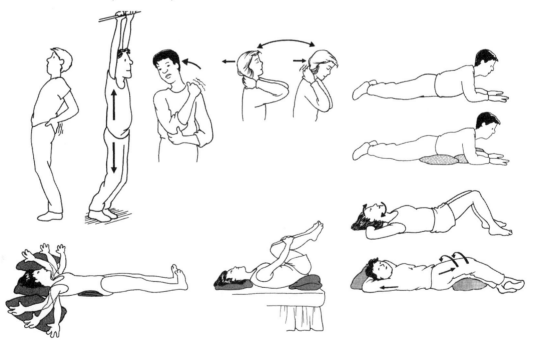

Figure 4.63

BEDTIME

Before Sleeping

If you've been sitting most of the evening, and/or if you tend to wake up stiff in the morning, take the time to lengthen out on your side, back, or stomach for a few minutes before going to sleep; do a few of the lengthening and release exercises detailed in the next chapter (see pp. 134–163).

Sleeping

◆ Avoid stressful sleeping positions (FIG. 4.64). Unsupported stomach lying, back lying, and side lying can strain the lower back and neck.

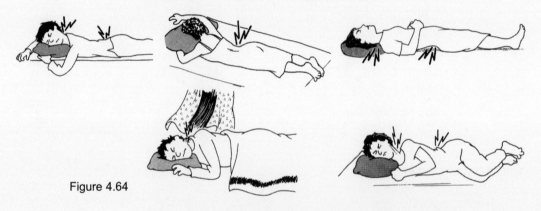

Figure 4.64

◆ Attempt using pillows and repositioning yourself to find the least stressful positions (FIG. 4.65).

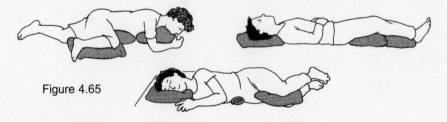

Figure 4.65

◆ Experiment to find the best pillow for your neck. There are a number of contoured or "cervical" pillows on the market today. It's always good if you can inspect them in person because they usually are not returnable items. Some pillows are shaped like a cylinder, while others are rectangular and offer contours and varying densities to support the neck and head. If it feels good, and you wake up feeling good, use it. If not, try different sized or shaped pillows.

In general, avoid extremes. Extremely soft and/or flat pillows will allow your head to drop backward when you lie on your back or down to the bed when you're side lying. If the pillow is too firm and/or fat, it will push your head too far forward when you lie on your back, or up toward the ceiling when you're side lying. Ideally, when you are on your back the pillow will support the slight forward curve of your neck; this is the "cylinder" portion of cervical pillows, and the back of the head will be supported so that it is not pushed forward or dropped backward. When side lying, the head and neck should be supported in neutral—that is, neither pushed up toward the ceiling nor dropped down toward the bed.

Choosing a Mattress

Once again, each individual's preference is a little different, so listen to your body and your past experience, and choose the kind of mattress that feels best to you. Keep in mind that mattresses that are too soft or too firm typically cause more strain on your neck and back. If you go the waterbed route, make sure it has a heater and is the firm variety. Futons generally do not have enough "spring" for most, but some back pain sufferers swear by them.

CHAPTER 5

Strategic Exercises

∨

RELEASE AND LENGTHENING EXERCISES

STRENGTHENING EXERCISES

AEROBIC EXERCISE

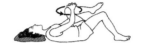

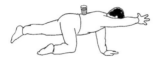

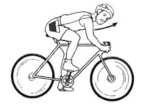

Muscular System

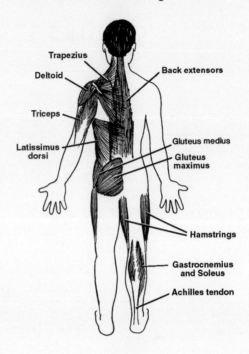

Trapezius
Deltoid
Triceps
Latissimus dorsi
Back extensors
Gluteus medius
Gluteus maximus
Hamstrings
Gastrocnemius and Soleus
Achilles tendon

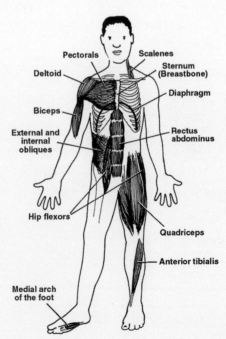

Pectorals
Deltoid
Biceps
External and internal obliques
Hip flexors
Medial arch of the foot
Scalenes
Sternum (Breastbone)
Diaphragm
Rectus abdominus
Quadriceps
Anterior tibialis

Performing a consistent exercise program can help to improve the condition and balance of your structural and electrical systems. This will make you less vulnerable to the physical, emotional, and mental stress in your life.

Exercise, like most things, can have either a good or a bad effect on your system, depending upon how well the exercise suits your specific needs and how you perform it. It is crucial that you become aware of what types of exercises your system needs and how to perform them correctly so that they are truly beneficial. The quality of your exercise performance is much more important than how much or how long you exercise.

All exercises are not equal; your exercise program should reflect both the immediate and long-range needs of your system. A balanced program will typically include a combination of the following types of exercises:

■ **Release and lengthening exercises** relax your electrical system, and they lengthen and decompress restricted, tense, and/or compressed areas of your structural system.

■ **Strengthening exercises** promote the strength, confidence, and stability of your structural and electrical systems.

■ **Aerobic exercises** promote endurance and weight loss. They can help make you less vulnerable to injury and chronic pain episodes.

The best way to achieve long-term pain control, improvement in your structure, and increased ability to function will be to combine a few elements from all three exercise groups. In general, most people will benefit by performing a few release and lengthening movements on a daily basis, strengthening exercise 2–4 times a week, and aerobic exercise 3–4 times a week.

Perhaps the hardest part of any exercise program besides getting it started is keeping it going when your home and/or work schedules get especially hectic. During these busier times, it is important to incorporate fitness into your everyday activities. Remember that simply using good breathing, alignment, and tone when sitting, walking, bending, and lifting can improve your fitness level!

CAUTION: IF YOU HAVE RECENTLY EXPERIENCED AN INCREASE IN YOUR PAIN, OR IF YOUR ENERGY IS LOW DUE TO A COLD, THE FLU, OR FOR SOME OTHER REASON, TREAT YOURSELF WITH THE RELIEF METHODS THAT SEEM TO WORK BEST FOR YOU (CHAPTER 2). YOU SHOULD PERFORM SOME OF THE RELEASE AND LENGTHENING EXERCISES, BUT YOU MAY WANT TEMPORARILY TO CURTAIL THE AEROBIC AND STRENGTHENING ASPECTS OF YOUR PROGRAM.

RELEASE AND LENGTHENING EXERCISES

What and Why

These exercises are similar to what most people typically think of as stretching exercises; however, they are subtly but significantly different in that they place the emphasis on relaxation and comfortable lengthening. By relaxing and lengthening various soft tissues that have become tense and/or shortened, you should find that you will feel less tension and pain and that you are able to move more efficiently. These exercises are rather restorative; that is, they require very little energy, and they can actually help you to release some of the compression, strain, and tension of daily life. They can be especially helpful when you've been in one position for too long, or if you've been performing a sustained, repetitive work or sports activity. By reversing the position you've been in, by minimizing strain and compression, and by simultaneously performing Cleansing and Calming Breaths, you can more readily bring your structure back toward a state of balance and harmony. These exercises can help your system to calm down, relax, and mellow out; they are especially helpful during those times when you feel tight, tense, anxious, stiff, stressed, tired, and/or whenever you are experiencing a recent increase in your pain.

General Principles
for Lengthening Tight, Tense Areas

Think of the area being lengthened as behaving like a spoiled child that needs help and encouragement. Your goal is to get the tissue to willingly relax and lengthen in the direction you wish it to go. The more you use force or attempt to hurry, the more the tissue will resist! If you hold your breath, are impatient, or adopt a negative attitude, the tissue will sense this and will resist giving in and letting go. If you stretch the tissue too quickly, too far, or too long, it will become irritated and will only fight you and resist your intentions. For best results, try to become aware of and emphasize the following:

■ Move slowly into the stretch position until you feel a comfortable lengthening sensation in the appropriate area. At this point, allow your breathing pattern (Cleansing and Calming Breaths) to produce a slight rise and fall in the part being lengthened. As you inhale, imagine a wave peaking in slow motion and let the wave cause the part you are stretching to buoy up and recoil slightly so that there is less pulling—that is, as you inhale, reduce the stretch a bit. As you exhale, picture the wave lowering and spreading out, and allow the part being stretched to release and lengthen back out to a comfortable degree (FIG. 5.1).

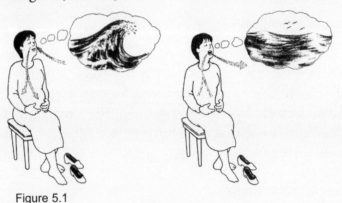

Figure 5.1

■ For each exercise described below, get into a comfortable position and sustain this pattern of breathing and stretching until the stretch sensation lessens. (This can be from 20 seconds up to three minutes.) You can move in and out of the stretch as much as you want as long as you move slowly and smoothly and allow the stretched part to relax in its lengthened position; in other words, no quick or forceful movements!

■ Seek comfort and pleasure during these exercises. Remember that you'll be able to stretch farther sooner if you don't force the stretch to the point of pain. Whenever you hit a barrier (feel discomfort or pain), reduce the amount of stretch and concentrate on relaxed breathing/imagery (see pp. 33–35).

■ Listen carefully to your body. In current research on flexibility exercises, there is no consensus on how many exercises to do or how long to hold each stretch. The literature recommends holding stretches until the stretch sensation lessens and performing enough exercises that the movement is easier than when you started. This suggests that every person is different and may require different amounts of repetition and hold time to achieve results.

■ A mild level of pain may occur during the stretch and remain up to three hours afterwards. However, by the end of the day or the next morning your pain should be no worse than it typically is. This assures you are making changes but not overdoing your stretching exercises.

Specific Exercises

Neck Release

Why: If you are feeling any tightness, tension, or pain in your neck and/or shoulders.

When: During your predictable periods of neck tightness, such as after sustained periods when the neck is held in a stationary position (A.M. rising; during/following typing, writing, reading, watching television, riding in a car, etc.). You can do this in a subtle manner if complete privacy is not possible. Do this until the stretch sensation lessens. Concentrate on relaxation, not repetition.

Beginning Position:

◆ Sit or stand tall.

◆ Turn one arm outward close by your side and relax it, letting the weight of it gently pull your shoulder downward and backward, toward your back
pockets (FIG. 5.2a).

◆ If increased stretch is desired, place your arm in a
stickup position with the chest up, shoulders down,
and hand placed further back than your elbow (FIG.
5.2b).

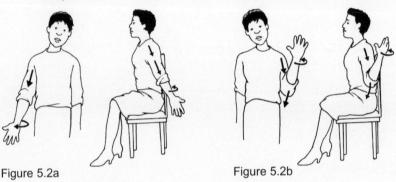

Figure 5.2a   Figure 5.2b

Movement:

◆ As you naturally exhale, elongate the side of your
neck by slowly tilting/turning toward the opposite
side. Pause when you feel a comfortable stretch and
hold until the stretch sensation lessens.

◆ Slowly move your neck in the following patterns,
pausing in these various positions when you feel a
comfortable/productive amount of stretch on the
side you're moving away from:

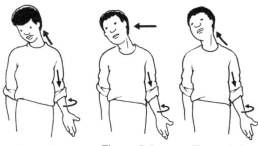

Figure 5.3   Figure 5.4   Figure 5.5

♦ Tilting right while turning right with the head slightly forward, you will feel stretch on the left side and back part of your neck and shoulder area (FIG. 5.3).

♦ Tilting right with the face straight ahead, you will feel stretch on the left side of your neck and the top of your shoulders (FIG. 5.4).

♦ Tilting right while turning right with the head slightly backward, you will feel stretch on the left side and front part of your neck and shoulders (FIG. 5.5).

CAUTION: IF YOU TILT BACK TOO FAR, YOU MAY FEEL AN UNCOMFORTABLE PRESSURE IN THE NECK AND/OR SHOULDER AREA ON THE SIDE YOU ARE TILTING TOWARD.

Alternate Methods:

♦ Rest the opposite hand across the collarbone and top of the shoulders—this assists in keeping the shoulder down while you move the head toward the opposite side (FIG. 5.6a).

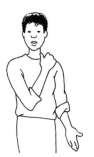

Figure 5.6a

♦ As above, support the "resting" hand by cupping the elbow with your opposite hand. The "resting" top hand can also be used to massage tight areas (FIG. 5.6b).

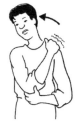

Figure 5.6b

◆ Tilt/Turn the head and neck to the left while your left hand gently pulls your right arm down and across behind your back (FIG. 5.6c).

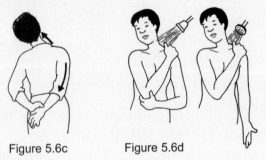

Figure 5.6c   Figure 5.6d

◆ Do this exercise in the shower—the warm, pulsing water can assist with pain relief and relaxation (FIG. 5.6d).

Note: Allow a relaxed breathing pattern to assist you in releasing the tension/tightness. Do not use force or maintain the head/neck in an uncomfortable part of the range! If you are uncomfortable, return to the starting position gently and in "slow motion." If one side is significantly tighter, spend more time (not force) on it, and release it more frequently.

Neck Straightening and Decompression

Why: This simple movement helps to decompress and straighten the neck, bringing the head into a more balanced position over the trunk. Besides producing better-looking posture, this repositioning helps decrease pain, muscle activity, and wear and tear on the joints and discs.

When: Same as for the Neck Release, but especially during activities that tend to cause the head to drop forward or stick out and forward (A.M. rising; during/following typing, writing, reading, watching television, riding in a car, etc.).

Beginning Position: This movement can be done while sitting, standing, walking, or lying on your back. (See pp. 27–29 for full explanation.)

Movement, Standing:

◆ Glide your head back over your chest.

◆ Look straight ahead and keep the head level, not looking up or down.

◆ Attempt to pull your chin in gently as far as possible without tensing up your shoulders or the front of your neck or throat. (Use your hand to help achieve this posture).

◆ Hold this position and consciously relax your breathing and muscles.

◆ Rest in this position as long as comfort allows.

◆ Imagine there are balloons gently pulling your head upward.

◆ Make sure you keep your muscles light and relaxed.

◆ Repeat this throughout the day (3–5 times) while in standing positions.

Movement, Standing Using a Wall (Fig. 5.7a):

◆ Place your feet about one foot away from the wall.

◆ Rest your upper back against the wall.

◆ Pull your head back with your chin tucked in so that your neck flattens out towards the wall. Keep your neck muscles light and relaxed.

◆ Hold this position for 20–60 seconds.

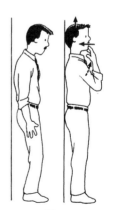

Figure 5.7a

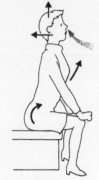

Figure 5.7b

Movement, Sitting (FIG. 5.7b):

◆ Reposition your pelvis as described on pages 52–53.

◆ If there is a neck rest on your chair, use it as you would use the wall in the position described above.

◆ Push through your arms to assist in lifting your chest wall and moving your lower back away from the backrest as your head and neck glide back.

Movement, Lying Position:

◆ Fold a towel to whatever size allows your head to stay level (FIG. 5.8a); avoid folding the towel so that it is too high or too low.

◆ Pull the towel so that your head and neck move with it into an even straighter, more lengthened position (FIG. 5.8b).

◆ Relax here and breathe for a few minutes (FIG. 5.8c). If you then want more of a lengthening feeling, you can pull the towel again to create more stretch.

◆ Use heat or cold in this position to assist in relief efforts.

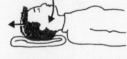

Figure 5.8a

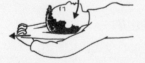

Figure 5.8b

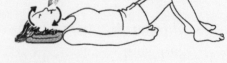

Figure 5.8c

Spinal Counter Rotation Exercise

Why: This is a whole-body exercise that can promote improved flexibility and general relaxation. It tends to lengthen the body out and allows for easier turning and reaching.

When: Whenever you feel tight, tense, stiff, angry, or depressed. If you do this in the morning, move extra slowly and support yourself with pillows. If done just before bedtime, this exercise may help to promote a better night's rest.

Beginning Position (FIG. 5.9a):

◆ Lie on your back on a firm but comfortable surface, with your hips and knees bent. Go barefoot or wear rubber sole shoes so that your feet do not slide on the surface.

◆ Begin with 1–2 slow, deep Cleansing Breaths. Rest your hands on your abdomen to assist with a deep diaphragm breath.

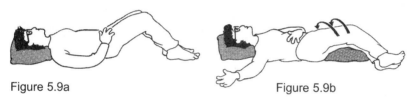

Figure 5.9a Figure 5.9b

Movement, Lower Trunk Phase (FIG. 5.9b):

◆ Allow gravity to lower your knees gently toward the left; allow your knees, pelvis, and lower back to relax so that gravity pulls them down toward the floor.

◆ If you feel stiff or tense about letting them go, place your hands on the outsides of your thighs for a little support, and perform the lowering motion to the rhythm of your natural breathing pattern—stop lowering your legs when you inhale, then allow further lowering as you exhale—and continue this pattern until the legs will go no further.

◆ If you feel a productive amount of stretch, rest in this end-range position until the stretch sensation lessens.

◆ If you feel discomfort, attempt to reduce or eliminate it by using your arms or pillows to block the range that sets off the pain. For example, if pain occurs with lowering your legs to the left, place your hand and/or a pillow on the floor under the outside of your left leg to limit the motion and support your legs so that you can totally relax. Over time, the leg and lower trunk should be able to roll further without causing tension or pain.

Movement, Neck and Arm Phase (FIG. 5.9c):

◆ Once you've reached a comfortable position of the lower trunk to the left, move your right arm slowly out to the side (9–11 o'clock) until you reach a comfortable stretch position.

◆ Turn your head and look toward your outstretched arm as long as you feel a comfortable lengthening sensation in the neck. If you feel no more than a comfortable amount of stretch in any area of your body, rest in this position.

◆ Take a few Cleansing and Calming Breaths, and hold in this position until the stretch sensation lessens.

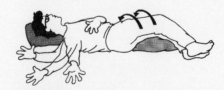

Figure 5.9c

◆ Slowly unwind from this position in the easiest way possible, moving one body part at a time (head, arm, leg, pelvis, etc.).

◆ If any discomfort occurs with the above sequence, attempt to reduce neck and/or arm pain by not going as far into the range. Placing a pillow under your arm will decrease the amount of stretch you feel and allow you to really let go.

Advanced Counter-Rotation/Elongation

When: If you felt like the preceding exercise was comfortable but gave you little or no stretch sensation.

Movement:

◆ Start by rolling completely onto your left side. Straighten out your top (right) leg at the knee and allow it to bend forward at the hip (placing a large pillow under the leg will be more comfortable) (Fig. 5.10a).

◆ Now "unwind" the top half of your body by raising your right arm from your side and reaching it slowly overhead in an up and backward direction. Stop raising your arm as you inhale; continue raising as you exhale. Support your right arm on pillows in any position where you feel a comfortable amount of lengthening; hold until the stretch sensation lessens (Fig. 5.10b).

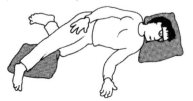

Figure 5.10a

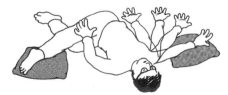

Figure 5.10b

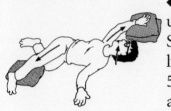

Figure 5.10c

♦ For a comfortable sustained stretch, place pillows under your outstretched arm and/or leg as needed. Support them up high enough so that you can totally relax the arm and leg without discomfort (FIG. 5.10c). As you become more flexible, you can gradually reduce the height of the pillows so that your arm and leg lower closer to the floor.

Knees to Chest: Slowly Rocking and Rolling

Why: This exercise can gently lengthen and relax the lower back and buttocks areas.

When: It may be especially helpful after sustained standing, walking, wearing high heels, reaching overhead, swimming, or after lying straight out on your stomach or back. This exercise is also helpful when you feel that your lower back is stiff from "holding" yourself tensely in any position, such as sitting, for a long time.

Beginning Position (FIG. 5.11a)*:* Same as for Spinal Counter Rotation exercise.

♦ Lie on your back on a firm but comfortable surface, with your hips and knees bent.

♦ Go barefoot or wear rubber-sole shoes so that your feet do not slide on the surface.

♦ Begin with 1-2 slow, deep Cleansing Breaths. Rest your hands on your abdomen to assist with a deep diaphragm breath.

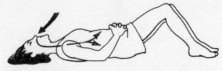

Figure 5.11a

Movement, Single Knee:

♦ Gently raise one knee up and grasp it by interlacing your fingers. Keep the arms relaxed and fully stretched out at first.

♦ Slowly pulling with your arms, allow the leg to move in circles (clockwise and counterclockwise) (FIG. 5.11b).

♦ Take Calming Breaths and occasional Cleansing Breaths. Repeat with the opposite leg.

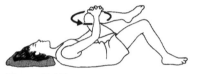 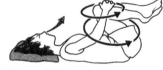

Figure 5.11b   Figure 5.11c

Movement, Both Knees:

♦ Proceed from the single–knee position to this one by pulling up the opposite leg.

♦ Repeat the slow, circular-movement pattern as described above (FIG. 5.11c).

♦ Take a few Cleansing Breaths and gently pull your knees toward your chest as you exhale.

Movement, Supported Knees to Chest:

♦ Starting in the beginning position, lift your buttocks up by pushing through both feet (try not to arch your back when lifting), and then pull a firm, thick pillow under your buttocks and tailbone (not your lower back) (FIG. 5.12a).

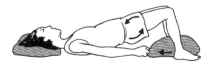

Figure 5.12a

♦ Once in the position illustrated, you should feel that your legs are totally relaxed and balanced (they should stay bent up without any effort).

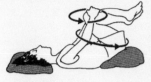

♦ Gently place your hands on the outside or top side of your legs and repeat the circular, rolling motion described above (FIG. 5.12b); gently pull the knees toward your chest as you exhale—there is no need for force!

Figure 5.12b

Pressups

Why: Pressups lengthen and decompress the spine.

When: Pressups may also be the quickest route to comfort when pain occurs after too much sitting, bending, or lifting.

Beginning Position (FIG. 5.13a):

♦ Lie on your stomach and prop yourself up on your elbows. Place a pillow under your abdomen if this is more comfortable.

♦ Shift your shoulders from side to side slowly and gently to relax, lengthen, and loosen the spine.

♦ Don't arch your neck up.

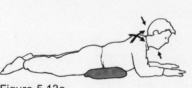
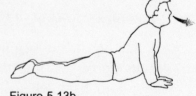

Figure 5.13a   Figure 5.13b

Movement (FIG. 5.13b):

♦ Take in a deep breath. As you exhale, push up with your arms and look straight ahead (don't arch the neck backward by looking up). Allow the chest to lift upright and the rest of the lower spine to sag and lengthen; keep your lower back relaxed and don't lift your pelvis up off the surface.

◆ Press up to the point of a comfortable lengthening and pressure sensation in your lower back. Pause there and take a relaxed breath—relax for about 3–5 seconds before lowering down to the starting position.

◆ Repeat this motion until it becomes easier.

Note: Gradually increase the range of your pressup according to comfort. Don't press up into a painful range; instead, stop when you feel a comfortable pressure. Commonly, the range of your pressup will increase with repetition.

Hands and Knees Rocking and Shifting

Why: This exercise moves the spine from a relatively rounded position to an arched one with no effects of weight bearing. It promotes improved flexibility and relaxation, and circulation to muscles, joints, and discs of the spine.

When: This is helpful when you've been stuck in one position or activity for too long and you feel stiff or tense. It's a nice way to get yourself moving in the morning or unwound at night.

Beginning Position: Rest on your hands and knees on a firm but padded surface.

Movement:

◆ Gently and alternately round and arch your spine through a small, comfortable range.

◆ As you round your back, gently pull your buttocks in and release your head and neck forward and down so you are looking toward your knees (FIG. 5.14a). Take a Cleansing Breath here.

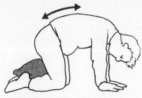
Figure 5.14a

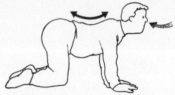
Figure 5.14b

◆ Now, allow your spine to sag in the middle as your buttocks stick out and as you lift your chest and head so you are looking forward (not up) (FIG. 5.14b). Take a Cleansing Breath here.

◆ Slowly repeat this movement from rounding to arching until the movement becomes easier.

Alternate Methods:

Figure 5.15

◆ From the beginning position, move your head and buttocks to the same side, much like a dog looking back at its tail. Take a Cleansing Breath here. Repeat to the opposite side (FIG. 5.15).

◆ From the beginning position, place a firm, fat pillow behind your knees. Gently rock backward so that you are "sitting" on the pillow and allow your spine to lengthen and round out, allowing your head to rest forward on your arms, the surface, or a pillow.

Take a few Cleansing Breaths in this position and rest for a moment (FIG 5.16a).

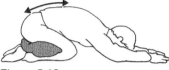

Figure 5.16a

◆ From this position walk your arms to the left to elongate the spine and the muscles on the right; take a few Cleansing Breaths and rest (FIG. 5.16b). Repeat, walking your arms to the right.

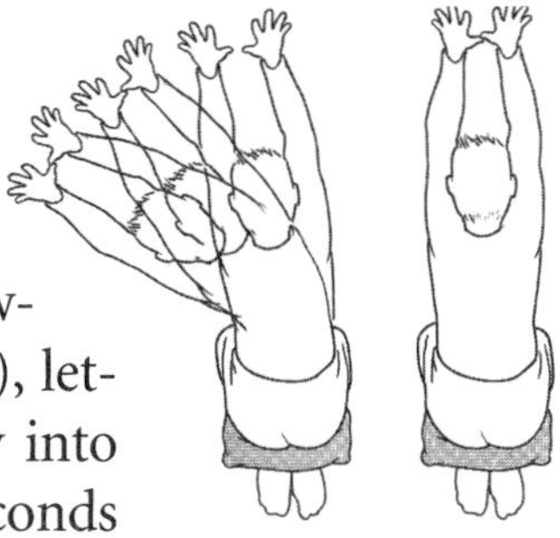

◆ From the heel-sitting position (FIG. 5.16a) slowly rock forward out over your arms (FIG. 5.17a), letting your lower spine sag smoothly and gently into the Pressup position (FIG. 5.17b). Pause a few seconds here and take a Cleansing Breath before returning to the starting position. Repeat going back and forth from heel sitting to the Pressup position until the movement gets easier.

Figure 5.16b

Note: This exercise combines elements of the Knee-to-Chest and the Pressup exercises; therefore it's an alternative to doing these two.

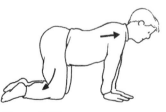

Figure 5.17a

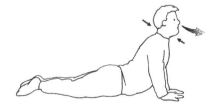

Figure 5.17b

Pelvic Rocking While Sitting

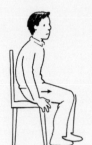

Figure 5.18a

Why: The basic movement described above can also be performed while sitting if you are unable to use the hands and knees position.

Beginning Position: Sitting on the edge of the chair.

Movement:

◆ Gently slump, allowing your spine to round from the bottom up (FIG. 5.18a).

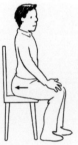

Figure 5.18b

◆ From this position rock your pelvis forward, allowing the lower spine to arch and your chest to lift (FIG. 5.18b).

◆ Repeat this movement until it feels easier.

Hamstrings Lengthening

Why: If your hamstrings are tight, they can exert a powerful pull on the pelvis, causing you to slump (especially during sitting and bending) and thereby resulting in a significant amount of compression and strain to your lower back.

When: It is probably best to work on lengthening hamstrings after they've warmed up (for example, after walking or cycling) or before and after sitting for long periods. You should not try to lengthen them first thing in the morning, when you're cold, or when you're tense!

CAUTION: YOU SHOULD NOT WORK ON LENGTHENING YOUR HAMSTRINGS IF YOU CAN ALREADY BRING YOUR LEG INTO THE RANGE ILLUSTRATED IN FIGURE 5.19 WITHOUT ROUNDING OUT YOUR LOWER BACK OR BENDING THE OPPOSITE LEG. (PROBLEMS CAN ARISE IF YOUR HAMSTRINGS ARE TOO LOOSE.) ALSO, DON'T STRETCH YOUR HAMSTRINGS IF YOU EXPERIENCE NERVE PAIN IN THE LEG WHILE ATTEMPTING TO PERFORM THESE EXERCISES.

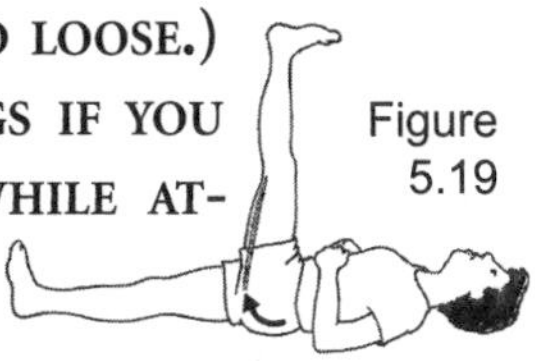

Figure 5.19

Beginning Position: Lie on your back with your legs straight. If this is uncomfortable, place a small folded towel or sheet under your lower back for support.

Movement:

◆ Bend up one leg with the foot flat on the floor. Lift up the opposite leg and interlace your fingers behind the thigh.

◆ While holding this position, slowly straighten the knee until you feel a comfortable pulling sensation behind the thigh or knee (FIG. 5.20a). Hold the leg in this lengthened position while maintaining a relaxed breathing pattern until the stretch sensation lessens.

◆ Repeat this exercise with each leg until you feel you are more mobile than when you started.

◆ If this doesn't feel like much of a pull, straighten the bent leg out on the floor to gain an increased pull (FIG. 5.20b).

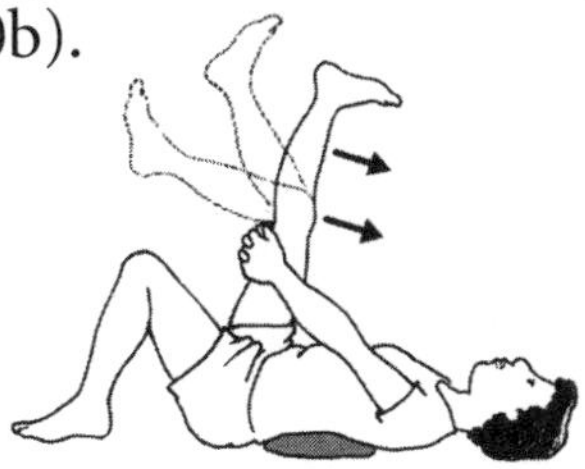

Figure 5.20a 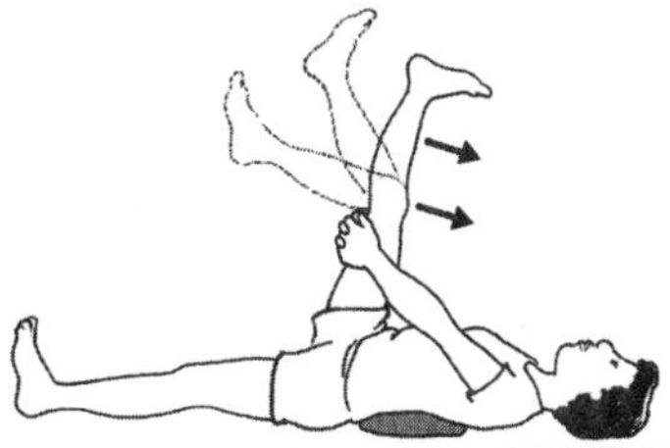   Figure 5.20b

Sustained Posterior Leg Lengthening with a Strap

Why: If your hamstrings are really tight, this method will allow you to maintain the lengthened position long enough and comfortably enough to make some real changes.

When: It is probably best to work on lengthening hamstrings after they've been warmed up (for example, after walking or cycling). You should not try to lengthen them first thing in the morning, when you're cold, or when you're tense!

Beginning Position: Lying on your back, bend a knee to your chest and wind a jump rope or long strap twice around the ball of your foot/shoe and twice around your wrist and hand so that it takes little effort to hold the rope or strap.

Movement:

◆ Slowly raise the leg until you feel a comfortable amount of stretch behind the thigh and/or calf. Keep the knee slightly bent (FIG. 5.21a).

◆ Raise both arms overhead and bend the knee as needed to find a balance point that takes little effort to maintain (FIG. 5.21b).

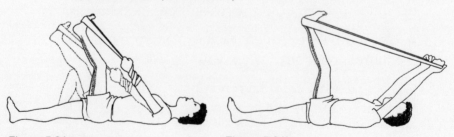

Figure 5.21a   Figure 5.21b

◆ Take both ends of the rope or strap in the hand opposite your raised leg. Allow your raised leg and arm to cross slightly over the midline of your body to produce a comfortable amount of stretch sensation to the outside of the calf, thigh, and pelvis (FIG. 5.22a).

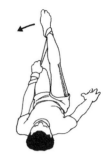

Figure 5.22a

◆ Maintain this stretch pattern until the stretch sensation lessens before returning to the middle position.

◆ Repeat enough times until the movement becomes easier.

◆ Now take both ends of the rope or strap in the other hand. Allow your raised leg and arm to move slightly to the outside to produce a comfortable amount of stretch sensation along the inside of the thigh (FIG. 5.22b).

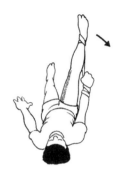

Figure 5.22b

◆ Maintain this stretch pattern until the stretch sensation lessens before returning to the middle position. Repeat until the movement becomes easier.

Note: It is crucial to maintain a relaxed breathing pattern during this exercise. If you are holding your breath or tensing up, the tissue won't lengthen.

Sitting Hamstrings Lengthening

Why: This method can be used as an alternative to the methods shown above.

When: This works well when you cannot stand up or lie down.

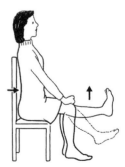

Beginning Position: Sit on the edge of a chair with a slight arch in your lower back (FIG. 5.23).

Figure 5.23

Movement:

◆ Without moving your spine, slowly straighten your knee and pull your toes toward your face (FIG. 5.23).

◆ Hold this position until the stretch sensation lessens; return to start position.

◆ Repeat with opposite leg.

Standing Hamstrings Lengthening

Why: This method can be used as an alternative to the methods shown above. This standing method may be the easiest way to lengthen your hamstrings without getting down on the floor. It also allows you to maintain the stretch with little effort.

When: This method is helpful when you've been sitting for too long or if the back of your legs feel tight or stiff.

Beginning Position: Stand at the bottom of the stairs using the wall and/or railing for support so that you are relaxed and standing up tall.

Movement:

◆ Keep your "standing" leg straight (but don't lock the knee), with the foot straight ahead. Raise the other leg up onto the second, third, or fourth step. Rest your heel on the step and move forward so that the bottom of your ankle is supported close to a 90-degree position. By standing up tall (keeping your chest up), you will feel a stretch in the area of the hamstrings (FIG. 5.24a). Hold this position until the stretch sensation lessens before switching legs.

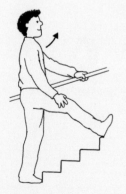

Figure 5.24a

◆ If you want more of a stretch, either raise your leg up to a higher step or lean forward out over the leg, keeping your chest up tall (don't bend down over the leg by slumping and dropping your chest!) (FIG. 5.24b).

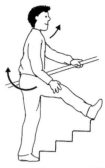

Figure 5.24b

◆ By keeping your feet straight ahead and twisting your arms and torso to the left and right, you will feel a more specific stretch to the inside and outside of your raised leg (FIG. 5.24 c and d).

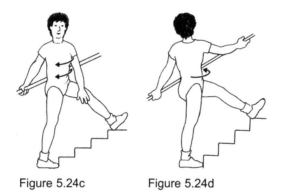

Figure 5.24c   Figure 5.24d

Alternate Methods: If you don't have access to stairs, a small stepstool, chair, sturdy box, etc., can be used to do this stretch.

Calf Lengthening

Why: Tight calf muscles may occur after running, wearing high heels or boots, and/or sustained sitting and bedrest. Calf tightness can result in pain and/or injury in the calf/foot itself. More commonly, it contributes to subtle tightness and inefficiency in the whole leg during walking, which may have a negative effect on your leg or back pain.

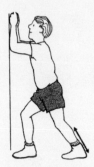

Figures 5.25a

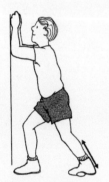

Figures 5.25b

When: Your calves are naturally tighter first thing in the morning. Let them stretch out naturally by means of slow, smooth walking. Calf Lengthening while standing should be done only after you've been up and around for a few hours. How frequently you do these exercises depends on how much your calves tend to tighten up. If you run, do aerobic dancing, wear high heels, etc., you should probably check for tightness before and after these activities, and lengthen your calves if they feel tight.

Beginning Position:

♦ Stand in front of a wall, counter, or tree.

♦ Place the leg to be stretched about two feet behind you. Bend the other leg and place it close to the wall, counter, or tree. Make sure both feet are facing straight ahead, not turned out! (Fig. 5.25a)

♦ If your foot tends to flatten out or roll inwards, place a magazine or towel just under the inside border of the foot being stretched (Fig. 5.25b).

Movement:

♦ Prop your arms on the wall and lean your hips forward, allowing the front leg to bend and keeping the rear leg straight back behind you with the heel on the ground. If your calves are tight, you will feel a definite pulling in your calf and/or Achilles tendon.

♦ Hold this position until the stretch sensation lessens while relaxing and breathing.

♦ To focus the stretch down to your lower calf toward your heel, bend the knee of your back leg slightly and maintain a comfortable lengthening sensation.

◆ Repeat the straight-leg and bent-knee positions with each leg until the motion feels easier.

Alternate Method: The following method is more aggressive and should be used if you didn't feel much stretch with the first method.

◆ Place the ball of your foot across the edge of a curb or bottom step. Place your other foot flat up on the curb or next step. Hold on and/or lean up against the railing or post for balance so that you are standing tall and relaxed.

◆ Allow your rear heel to lower to produce a comfortable lengthening sensation. By bending the knee slightly, you will feel the stretch move lower down toward the heel. Do not lock the knee straight (FIG. 5.26).

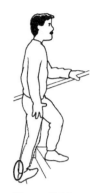

Figure 5.26

◆ Relax in the stretch position until the stretch sensation lessens and repeat until the motion feels easier.

Back Lying Hip Flexor Stretch

Why: If the hip flexors are tight, they can exert a forward pull on the pelvis and lower back, which results in increased strain. This results in the lower abdomen being pulled forward, which has a weakening effect on your lower abdominal muscles (FIG. 5.27).

When: This method is helpful when you've been sitting too long or if the front of your hips feels tight or stiff.

Beginning Position:

◆ Place a pillow on the end of your bed and sit near the edge.

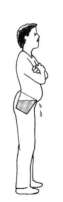

Figure 5.27

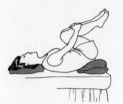

Figure 5.28a

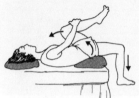

Figure 5.28b

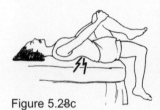

Figure 5.28c

◆ Lower yourself onto your back, bringing both knees up toward your chest to flatten out your lower back (FIG. 5.28a).

Movement:

◆ Hold one knee firmly to your chest while you slowly lower the other leg down (FIG. 5.28b). You will feel pulling across the top of the hip, thigh, and/or knee of your lowered leg. Make sure to keep the opposite leg bent firmly to your chest so that your back stays flat. If it gets pulled forward at all, you may not feel any tightness in the down leg, and you may hurt your back (FIG. 5.28c).

◆ Take in a deep breath and as you exhale continue to relax the leg so that it lowers down as far as possible. Do not allow the leg to move out to the side. Let it relax down and lengthen until the stretch sensation lessens.

◆ Assess each leg separately and treat each appropriately; that is, if both legs feel and/or appear tight, lengthen them both; if only one is tight, work only on it.

CAUTION: WHEN SWITCHING LEGS, BRING BOTH KNEES TOWARD YOUR CHEST FIRST (FIG. 5.28a), THEN LOWER THE SECOND LEG. DO NOT LET BOTH LEGS HANG OFF THE EDGE OF THE BED AT THE SAME TIME.

Standing Hip Flexor Stretch

Why: If you are unable to do the Back Lying Hip Flexor Stretch.

When: This move is helpful when you've been sitting too long or if the front of your hips feels tight or stiff.

Beginning Position: Stand alongside a chair or counter and place your hand up on the counter or chair for support.

Movement:

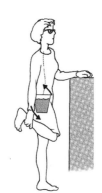

Figure 5.29a

◆ Bend the hip and knee of your outside leg behind you so that you can grab it around the ankle (FIG. 5.29a).

◆ Now slowly lower your thigh to straighten your hip as much as possible. If tight, your thigh will tend to stick out sideways and/or will be difficult to straighten and/or your back will arch (FIG. 5.29b). If this happens, reduce the amount of stretch. You should feel only a comfortable lengthening at the front of the hip and/or thigh.

◆ Maintain a level pelvis as you lower the thigh—do not allow your abdomen to stick out or your back to arch; if this happens, tense up your buttocks and lower abdominal muscles to keep your pelvis level.

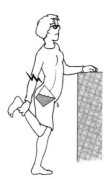

Figure 5.29b

◆ Maintain the stretch until the sensation lessens and repeat as described above.

Alternate Movement: If this movement produces discomfort, or if you feel like your back is arching, decrease the stretch by supporting your leg on a chair behind you (FIG. 5.30).

Overhead Bar Lengthening

Why: This is an easy way to undo some of the compressive and shortening effects of daily life. By adding a few moments of

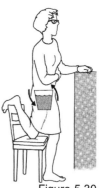

Figure 5.30

this exercise from time to time, you can assist in maintaining the optimal length of your structure and gain a sense of comfort and relaxation. It's especially good for loosening up the shoulder area and lengthening and decompressing the lower back.

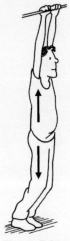

Figure 5.31a

When: The beginning and end of the day may be the times when your body would most appreciate a few moments of lengthening. If you place the bar in a doorway near your bedroom or bathroom, you may be more apt to use it when getting up or turning in.

Beginning Position: Keep your feet on the ground with your knees slightly bent for best results (FIG. 5.31a). (If you lift your feet up, your trunk muscles will contract and you'll lose the decompression effect.)

Movement:

♦ Take enough weight through your arms to direct the decompression to your lower back (if you simply "hang" from your arms, you will feel a strong pull/stretch through your arms and not much decompression to your lower back). Allow your legs to relax a bit to increase your traction. If your hands become uncomfortable or slippery, wear gloves or put padded foam around the bar.

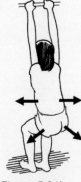

Figure 5.31b

♦ By simply holding onto the bar, you may feel a gentle lengthening and decompression. Increase the benefits of this exercise by allowing your pelvis to sway slowly in different directions, and experiment with moving your feet and hands in various positions to exert lengthening to the front, back, and either side of your trunk and pelvis (FIG. 5.31b).

♦ Perform some Cleansing Breaths and feel how this lengthened position helps fully ventilate your body.

STRENGTHENING EXERCISES

Many individuals who experience neck or back pain for longer than a few months lose a significant amount of strength. As the body loses strength, it loses stability, and this loss of stability makes it easier for you to become stressed (physically and emotionally) by your daily activities, thus making it easier to set off pain symptoms. Therefore, strengthening exercises can assist you in performing your activities in a more relaxed and efficient manner, and can decrease your pain.

As with release and lengthening exercises, when you do the strengthening exercises described below, your emphasis should be on the quality of your performance (maintaining balanced alignment and relaxed breathing). The recommendation is to perform at least 20 repetitions to build endurance of muscle and reinforce correct movement patterns. If your intent is to focus on strength development, then allow the lowering phase of the contraction to be slower (4–6 seconds) than the raising phase of the contraction (two seconds). If you're doing isometric strengthening, start by holding the contraction 5–10 seconds and work up to 45–60 seconds.

STRENGTHENING EXERCISES
USING BODY WEIGHT

Abdominal Strengthening

Abdominal strengthening is definitely important in the prevention and healing of back and neck injuries. The abdominals support the spine and pelvis from the front and sides. They work somewhat like guide wires, along with the extensor muscles of the back, to provide movement and to stabilize the spine in a relatively neutral, lengthened position. Therefore, the emphasis while strengthening the abdominals should be on performing smooth, controlled movements and on maintaining the spine in relatively low-stress, lengthened positions.

Unfortunately, many of the ways that people perform abdominal strengthening can actually aggravate low back and neck problems. The emphasis should not be on high-speed repetition or forceful movements where the spine is compressed and rounded.

▲ Here are some good moves to strengthen your abdominals more efficiently and safely:

Lower Abdominal Isometric

Why: Lower abdominal strengthening will help to support your spine (like a girdle) and prevent injury to it. It is especially important to have strong lower abdominal muscles when doing any type of exercise or activity. This exercise is sometimes called a pelvic tilt.

Beginning Position: Lie on your back with knees bent. As this exercise becomes easier, straighten your legs out on the floor.

Movement (FIG.5.32):

◆ Lift your lower abdomen up and in while maintaining a relaxed breathing pattern; your lower abdomen should stay relatively flat and should not protrude.

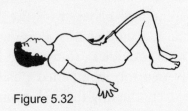

Figure 5.32

◆ At the same time, the lower back should flatten slightly towards the floor so that the spine is in a more neutral position (i.e., midway between rounded and arched). This should be a comfortable position for your spine.

◆ Initially attempt this isometric for 5–10 seconds at a time, progressing up to 45–60 seconds; continue breathing in a normal manner.

◆ If you're having difficulty pulling your abdomen in, place your hands below your navel and think of pulling in away from your hands.

Alternate Methods:

◆ As you gain control in this position, attempt the isometric for up to 60 seconds while standing, walking, sitting, or during any activity (FIG. 5.33).

◆ Think of actually lifting the weight of the upper body up off your lower back by gently pulling the abdominals up.

◆ The more your abdominals learn to work this way, the more you should be able to relax the front of the neck, and the more natural it will become to do the exercise throughout the day.

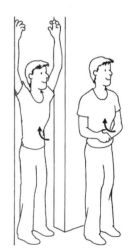

Figure 5.33

Abdominal Isometric with Leg Movements:

Why: These exercises strengthen the muscles in the front of the hip, knee, abdomen, and lower back. Besides strengthening, they can teach you how to keep your spine and pelvis stable while you move your legs.

Beginning Position:

◆ Lie on your back, with legs bent up and feet flat on the surface.

◆ Perform the isometric as described above (FIG. 5.32). Place your hands over your lower abdomen and pelvis to assist in giving you feedback—your abdomen should remain relatively flat and should not protrude.

◆ Your lower back should remain relatively flat against the surface, not pulling up and forward as you perform the following progression of movements:

Movement—Single-leg extension with the opposite leg bent and foot planted on the floor:

◆ Slowly extend the leg out straight as long as your back and abdomen remain comfortable and stable in the alignment described above; slowly move the leg back and forth from bent to straight position (FIG. 5.34a).

◆ The closer the leg is to the floor, the more difficult the exercise; therefore, if you're straining, don't extend the leg so straight or so low to the ground (FIG. 5.34b).

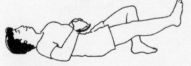
Figure 5.34a

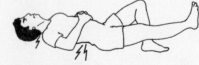
Figure 5.34b

◆ If you find this easy, extend the leg straight and about one inch off the floor, with your lower back neutral and your abdomen flat.

Movement—Double-leg slide:

◆ Slowly slide both legs out in a straight position with your feet on the floor (FIG. 5.35). The straighter your legs get, the harder you have to work to keep your back from arching and your abdomen flat.

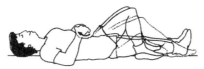

Figure 5.35

◆ Continue straightening your legs until they are resting straight on the surface and the feet are pulled up off the floor; return to the starting position one leg at a time (attempting to slide both legs simulta-neously is usually too stressful).

Movement—Single-leg extension with both legs bent and feet up off the surface:

◆ Bend both knees up to your chest using your arms; then slowly release, using your abdominals to main-tain your legs-bent, feet-up position (FIG. 5.36a).

◆ Slowly extend one leg out while keeping the back flat and the other leg bent. If you can control this comfortably, repeat the movement several times, then try it on the other side (FIG. 5.36b).

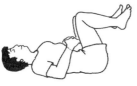 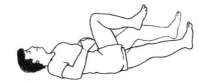

Figure 5.36a   Figure 5.36b

Movement—Straight Leg Raising (SLR)

(A) **SLR**—OPPOSITE LEG BENT (FIG. 5.37):

◆ Press your fingers against the sides of your lower abdomen and pull up and in so that your lower back remains in neutral alignment.

◆ Keep your trunk and pelvis stable; don't let them move as you slowly lift the straight leg to a 50-70 degree angle.

◆ Hold the leg up for about five seconds before lowering it slowly to the ground.

◆ Make sure to keep the abdomen firm and the back flat against the floor as you lift and lower the leg.

◆ Practice relaxed breathing throughout the sequence.

◆ Repeat 5-20 times with each leg.

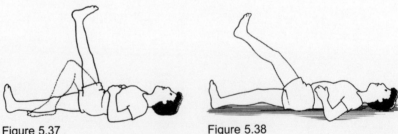

Figure 5.37   Figure 5.38

(B) **SLR**—OPPOSITE LEG STRAIGHT (FIG. 5.38): This method is more advanced than the above exercise.

◆ As before, tighten up your abdominal muscles and flatten your back slightly against the floor.

◆ Maintain this posture and keep this area from moving as you lift and lower one leg.

◆ Keep the other leg flat, relaxed, and unmoving.

◆ Repeat 5-20 times for each leg.

Partial Curl-ups (FIG. 5.39):

Why: These exercises will help to strengthen abdominals.

Beginning Position: Lie on your back with knees bent and feet on the floor or lower legs resting on a chair.

Movement—Straight Curl-ups:

◆ Place the hands loosely behind the head to support its weight (without pulling it forward).

◆ Keep the elbows back and outward (so they do not pull in front of the shoulders).

◆ Lift and lead the motion with your chest, allowing the head to stay back in line with the chest. As you curl up, concentrate on bringing the bottom of your breastbone and your navel closer together— you should automatically perform a lower abdominal isometric (pelvic tilt) as you lift.

◆ Maintain the partial curl-up position about 3–5 seconds before slowly lowering. As you lower, make sure your spine stays flat on the floor.

◆ Practice relaxed breathing throughout the sequence: exhale as you curl up and inhale as you lower.

◆ Repeat 5–20 times.

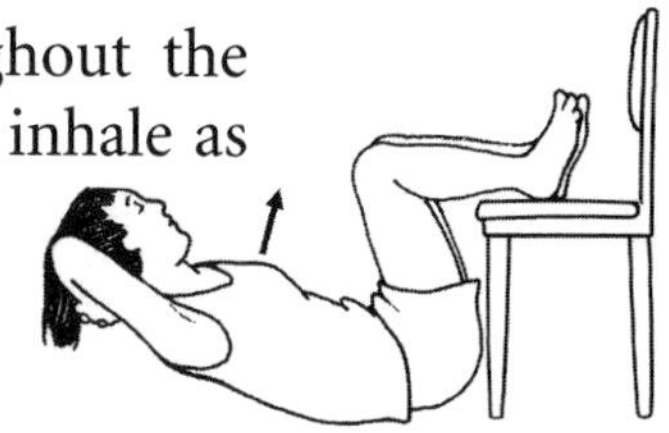

Figure 5.39

Movement—Rotational Curl-ups:

◆ Perform the same movement as above, but twist as you pull up so that your left armpit moves toward your right knee or your right armpit moves toward your left knee (Fig. 5.40a).

◆ Once again, keep the elbows relatively outward to the side and the head back in the hands as you pull up and over to one side.

◆ Hold the curl-up for 3–5 seconds and repeat 5–20 times.

◆ You can vary this exercise by lifting and pulling the knee toward the opposite armpit as you lift up and across with your trunk (Fig. 5.40b). Do this exercise 5–20 times with each leg.

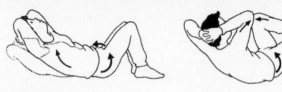

Figure 5.40a   Figure 5.40b

Curl-ups with Legs Up (Fig. 5.41):

Why: If the previous exercise causes discomfort to your lower back.

Beginning Position: Bring both knees to your chest and stretch them there for a moment with your hands to flatten out your back against the floor. As you let go of the legs with your hands, the abdominal muscles have to contract to maintain the flat-back position.

Movement:

◆ Repeat the Partial Curl-up motion of the chest and head. Simultaneously lift the tailbone up further off the floor so that the base of the breastbone and the navel move closer together.

◆ Hold for 3–5 seconds while you breathe. Lower down slowly.

◆ Relax and repeat 5–20 times.

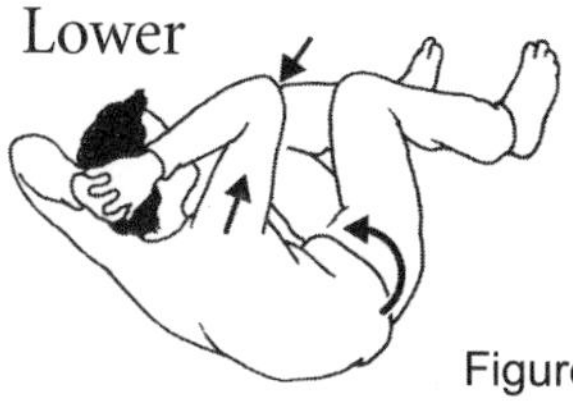

Figure 5.41

Alternate Method for Abdominal Strengthening:

If your low back or neck pain is made worse by attempting the preceding sit-ups, you can still strengthen your abdominals isometrically during standing and walking (see FIG. 5.33). Simply pull your lower abdomen up and in, away from the waistband of your clothing, while you maintain a relaxed breathing pattern. Attempt this flattening of your lower abdominal area as you stand and walk. Relaxed breathing during this exercise will help to make it more natural and will allow you to maintain it longer, for example, 20 seconds up to one minute at a time. This method of strengthening can be done during regular daily activities, such as A.M. /P.M. bathroom times, walking, waiting for elevators, etc.

▼ Bad Moves when doing abdominal exercises:

▼ Avoid doing curl-ups or bent-knee sit-ups if they result in increased low back or leg pain. If your pain is aggravated by sitting or bending, it is best to avoid these and to strengthen your abdomen by performing lower abdominal isometrics in back-lying, standing, and walking positions.

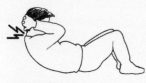

Figure 5.42

▼ Avoid bending or pulling your head and neck forward in front of the chest. When doing abdominal exercises, people often forcefully pull on the back of the head with their hands. This strains the neck, encourages poor posture, and reduces the workload to your abdominal muscles (FIG. 5.42).

▼ Avoid doing straight-leg sit-ups or hooking your feet under furniture if you tend to arch your lower back as you pull up. Both of these methods work the hip flexor muscles, which allows the abdominals to "take a break" (FIG. 5.43).

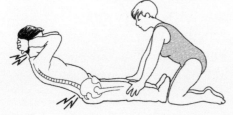
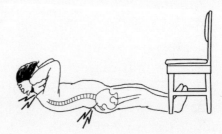

Figure 5.43

▼ Avoid going fast. Going fast means you're using momentum to do the exercise, which is less effective for strengthening. Going fast also makes it much easier to injure or at least aggravate your neck and lower back because of the pumping and compression that occur at higher rates of speed.

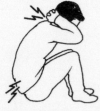

Figure 5.44

▼ Avoid attempting to pull up more than one-third of the way. The abdominals work very hard through the first one-third of the range; after that, you tend to pull in the hip muscles, and you're simply increasing compression and strain to your lower back and neck (FIG. 5.44).

▼ Avoid dropping back down from the sit-up position. The lowering phase is just as important for strengthening as the sitting-up phase. Therefore, lower yourself smoothly and slowly back to the starting position.

▼ Avoid holding your breath when performing abdominal exercises. Holding the breath puts extra strain on your spine, which may cause pain. It is best to exhale as you raise up and contract your abdominals and inhale as you are lowering back down.

Neck Strengthening

Isometric Neck Strengthening

Why: These exercises will be helpful if your neck feels weak—as if you can't hold your head up for very long without getting tired.

Beginning Position: Position yourself in your best sitting or standing posture. Make sure your head is balanced upright and level over your chest, not forward or with the chin sticking out or hanging down. No movement of the head should occur with these exercises. Hold each position gently for 5–60 seconds while maintaining a relaxed breathing pattern.

(A) BACK OF NECK: Place your hand around the back and base of your head; pull forward with your hand, simultaneously pulling back and in with your neck so that the head stays still and in good alignment (FIG. 5.45a).

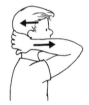

Figure 5.45a

(B) SIDE OF NECK: Move your hand around to the side (over your ear). Repeat the isometric sequence described in (a) in a sideways direction. Repeat this on the opposite side (FIG. 5.45b).

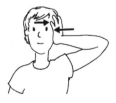

Figure 5.45b

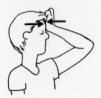

Figure 5.45c

(C) FRONT OF NECK: Strengthen the front of the neck in this same isometric manner by bringing your hand around to the front and pushing against the forehead while maintaining the head in a good neutral posture (FIG. 5.45c).

Head Lifting Exercise

Why: It is important to strengthen the front of your neck if you have difficulty lifting your head up from a reclining position.

Beginning Position: Lie on your back with your head supported on a relatively low, flat pillow. Perform Neck Straightening and Decompression (see pp. 27–29).

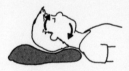

Figure 5.46

Movement (FIG. 5.46): Begin to lift the head, keeping the chin in and leading with your forehead so that you feel you have lifted ⅓–½ of its weight up off the surface. Hold 5–10 seconds in this position while maintaining a relaxed breathing pattern. Lower your head and release slowly. Repeat 3–5 times.

Back and Hip Strengthening Exercises

Hands and Knees Reaching

Why: This exercise strengthens the extensor muscles along the back of the body, including the thigh, buttocks, back, shoulders, and neck. It teaches your spine how to be stable, and it will improve your balance as well. These exercises are a good follow-up to the abdominal and neck strengthening exercises.

Beginning Position (FIG. 5.47a):

◆ Get into a hands-and-knees position. Keep your knees pelvic-width apart and your hands shoulder-width apart.

◆ Turn your arms slightly outward and position the wrists so they are comfortable.

◆ Keep your head and neck in a straight line with the rest of your back—in a flattened contour, not arched up or hanging down.

◆ Keep your lower back in whatever is its most re-laxed, neutral alignment (not rounded or sagging).

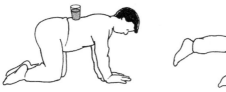

Figure 5.47a   Figure 5.47b

Movement:

◆ Pretend that there is a cup of water sitting in the middle of your back. Move in such a way that you keep the water level and tranquil throughout the re-mainder of this exercise—don't jar or spill it!

◆ Shift your weight to the left leg and slowly extend the right leg behind you so that it is fairly straight. Do not allow your pelvis and back to tip or twist (FIG. 5.47b).

◆ Hold your leg straight for 3–10 seconds before re-turning it as smoothly as possible.

◆ Repeat 5–10 times with each leg.

◆ Reach your right arm in front of you to the same level as your back—keep it in a thumbs-up position. Keep your head, neck, and back in a relaxed, neutral alignment—no arching, looking up, twisting, or straining—just relaxed reaching (FIG. 5.47c).

◆ Repeat 5–10 times with each arm.

◆ Combine arm and opposite-leg reaching patterns (FIG. 5.47d). Raise the arm and leg only as high as you can control without wobbling. Work toward being able to raise them so they are level with the back. Hold 3–10 seconds. Repeat 5–10 times on each side.

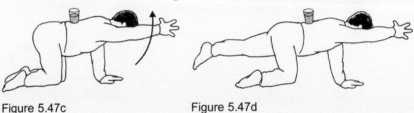

Figure 5.47c   Figure 5.47d

Stomach Lying Extension

Why: These exercises are similar to Hands and Knees Reaching in terms of why and how, so there is no need to do them both. Do the one you prefer. This exercise will help to develop stronger back muscles, hips, and shoulders.

Beginning Position: Lie on your stomach and rest your forehead on the backs of your hands or turn your head to the side. If your neck feels "cranked" or strained, place a flat pillow under your upper chest so that your head and neck can rest over the top comfortably. It may also be necessary to place a firm, flat pillow under your abdomen to assist in keeping the lower back from arching uncomfortably (FIG. 5.48).

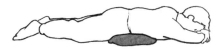

Figure 5.48

Movement:

◆ Perform a smooth, gentle pelvic tilt (FIG. 5.49a) so that your groin pushes into the pillow or floor and your back flattens out. Maintain the pelvic tilt and a relaxed breathing pattern while you perform the following:

◆ Single Leg Lifts: Lift your right leg up 2–4 inches only (FIG. 5.49b). Hold 3–10 seconds. Lower slowly and repeat 5-10 times. Repeat with the other leg.

◆ Single Arm Lifts: While keeping your head and neck relaxed, raise up one arm 2–4 inches in a straight-forward, thumbs-up direction. (FIG. 5.49c). Hold 3–5 seconds. Lower slowly and repeat 5-10 times. Repeat with the other arm.

◆ Arm and Leg Lifts: Lift your arm and opposite or same leg in the pattern described above (FIG. 5.49d). Hold 3–5 seconds and repeat 5-10 times. Repeat on each side.

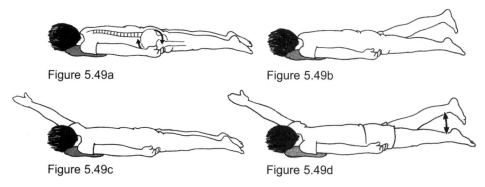

Figure 5.49a

Figure 5.49b

Figure 5.49c

Figure 5.49d

Bridging

Why: This exercise can strengthen abdominals, buttocks, back, and thighs. This may assist you to stand taller, get up out of a low chair, or climb stairs more easily.

Double Leg Bridging:

Beginning Position: Begin with a pelvic tilt to flatten your lower back against the floor (FIG. 5.50a).

Movement:

◆ Gently tighten your lower abdominal region and buttocks and roll the pelvis backward to smoothly lift it up off the floor; continue lifting (one vertebra at a time, like the links of a chain) until your pelvis and lower back are elevated above the floor (FIG. 5.50b).

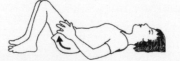
Figure 5.50a

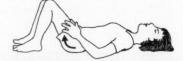
Figure 5.50b

◆ At the top of your lift, maintain a flat back and straight-line posture.

◆ Tighten your buttocks underneath you as you lift higher. Avoid arching your lower back (FIG. 5.51). Hold at the top for about five seconds while maintaining a relaxed breathing pattern.

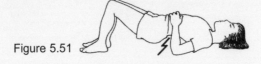
Figure 5.51

◆ Slowly lower—rolling down one vertebra at a time, starting with the upper vertebra and ending with your tailbone.

◆ Repeat 5–20 times.

Single Leg Bridging:

Beginning Position: Begin the same as in the Double Leg Bridge.

Movement:

◆ Once in the bridge-up position, imagine that there is a cup of water sitting atop your left knee. Attempt to slowly, smoothly shift your weight to the left leg so that you can lift the right leg and straighten the knee (FIG. 5.52). Attempt to do this without shaking or tilting, which would tend to spill the imaginary cup of water.

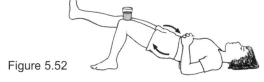

Figure 5.52

◆ Alternate lifting your left and right legs 5–20 times. Concentrate on not moving or tipping your pelvis. Make sure to maintain a relaxed breathing pattern throughout the exercise.

Side Bridging

Why: To improve overall posture by promoting strength, stability, and endurance of the side trunk, shoulder, and hip muscles.

Beginning Position: Start by lying on your side propped up on your elbow with knees bent and ears, shoulders, hips, and heels in line with each other (FIG. 5.53a).

Movement:

♦ Find neutral alignment of the lower back and elongate chest and head. Lower your bottom shoulder toward the floor; maintain this position as you raise your pelvis to the height of your shoulders, balancing on your knees and elbow (FIG. 5.53b).

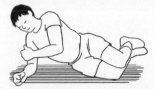   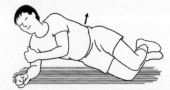

Figure 5.53a   Figure 5.53b

♦ Hold at the top for about five seconds while maintaining a relaxed breathing pattern.

♦ Repeat 5-20 times on each side.

Advanced:

♦ Start as above except with knees straight instead of bent; keep ears, shoulders, hips, knees, and heels in line with each other (FIG 5.54a).

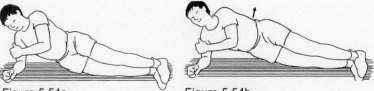

Figure 5.54a   Figure 5.54b

♦ Find neutral alignment of the lower back and elongate your chest and head. Lower your bottom shoulder toward the floor; maintain this position as you raise your pelvis to the height of your shoulders, balancing on your feet and elbow (FIG. 5.54b).

◆ Hold at the top for about five seconds while maintaining a relaxed breathing pattern.

◆ Repeat 5–20 times on each side.

Sideways Hip Strengthening

Why: The muscles that these exercises strengthen provide stability for the hip, pelvis, and lower back. If weakened, these muscles will allow increased side-to-side wobbling during standing and walking, resulting in increased strain.

Sideways Hip Strengthening—Outer Thigh:

Beginning Position: Lie on your side and support your head and neck comfortably on your hand or on pillows. Find neutral alignment of your spine. Place your top arm in front to keep you from rolling forward or backward off your side.

Movement:

◆ Rotate the top leg outward so the kneecap moves toward the ceiling and then lift the top leg (with knee straight) up no higher than illustrated (FIG. 5.55).

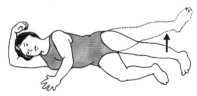

Figure 5.55

Pause 2–5 seconds before lowering smoothly.

◆ Repeat 5–20 times.

Sideways Hip Strengthening—Inner Thigh:

Beginning Position: Get in the same position as above but with the top leg bent and resting forward.

Movement:

◆ Lift the bottom leg straight up toward the ceiling so that at least the lower portion of the leg lifts up off the floor (FIG. 5.56). Hold 3–5 seconds before lowering smoothly.

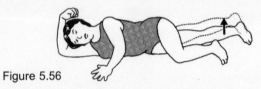

Figure 5.56

◆ Repeat 5–20 times on each side.

Standing Leg Lifts

Why: These exercises strengthen all the major muscles in the legs. By focusing on your head, trunk, and pelvis and maintaining them in their best neutral alignment, you will also strengthen the muscles that hold you in good posture, and you will help "teach" the muscles to hold you in good posture automatically. Because you are standing, these exercises also tend to improve your balance and coordination.

Beginning Position (for all these exercises):

◆ Stand with your head, trunk, and pelvis in their best alignment.

◆ Use doorways or counters to help you maintain your balance. It is most important to maintain good alignment, so attempting to let go of your arm support and losing your balance is a bad move.

◆ As your strength and balance improve, you can begin withdrawing your arm support by reducing your hold to one hand, one finger, etc.

◆ Finally, if possible, move away from supporting surfaces to do the exercises.

Movement (for all these exercises):

◆ Maintain relaxed breathing. If this exercise is too difficult for you at this time, you'll tend to hold your breath and tense up. If that happens, try to improve your strength with other exercises described in this section, then come back to this exercise and see if you can do it without holding your breath.

◆ Be sure to move the legs slowly and smoothly; this takes more strength and runs less risk of irritating your pain.

◆ Don't lift the legs so high that they pull your head, trunk, or pelvis out of alignment.

◆ Repeat 5–20 times with each leg.

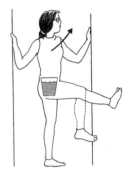

Figure 5.57

Forward Leg Raise—Knee Bent or Straight:

▲ *Good Moves:* Emphasize keeping your head and chest up tall! Only lift the leg as high as you can while maintaining this upright alignment (FIG. 5.57).

▼ *Bad Moves:* If not controlled, these movements will tend to pull the chest down, round the spine, and drop the head forward (FIG. 5.58).

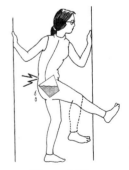

Figure 5.58

Backward Leg Raise—Knee Bent or Straight:

▲ *Good Moves:* Start out by pulling in your lower abdomen so your pelvic bowl is tipped relatively up and back under you. Keep your head in neutral with your eyes straight ahead. Move the leg back and stop before your pelvis starts tipping forward. The range should not be any further than that pictured if the exercise is done with pelvic control (FIG. 5.59).

▼ *Bad Moves:* If not controlled, these movements will tend to overarch the neck and low back areas, causing the chin and lower abdomen to stick out in a weak abdominal pattern (FIG. 5.60). This will occur if you try to move the leg too far back.

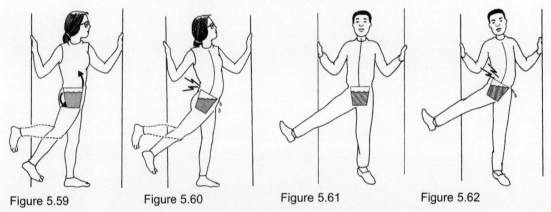

Figure 5.59   Figure 5.60   Figure 5.61   Figure 5.62

Sideways Leg Raising—Leg Straight:

▲ *Good Moves:* Keep your head, trunk, and pelvis vertically aligned and facing straight ahead. Raise the leg only as far as you can before any tipping or twisting occurs (FIG. 5.61).

▼ *Bad Moves:* Don't tip and tilt the trunk sideways; don't twist the pelvis and spine (FIG. 5.62).

Calf Raises:

▲ *Good Moves:* Keep your pelvis level by lightly tensing your lower abdomen and buttocks (see pp. 71–72). Smoothly raise up on your toes and lower. Maintain good foot and leg alignment (FIG. 5.63).

▼ *Bad Moves:* Avoid tipping your pelvis forward with your lower abdomen sticking out; avoid wobbling, jerky motion; avoid dropping quickly down to your heels; avoid splayed feet or feet too close together (FIG. 5.64).

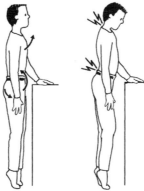

Figure 5.63   Figure 5.64

Squat Shifting

Why: This exercise is great for strengthening the legs and improving your balance, and it can help you to improve your squatting ability.

Beginning Position: Stand tall and move your feet wider than shoulder-width apart.

Movement:

◆ Partially squat down so that your knees are bending right over the tops of your feet (FIG. 5.65a).

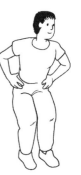

Figure 5.65a

◆ Begin to shift your weight slowly in a clockwise direction, moving your pelvis and trunk as far as possible over your feet in all directions: forward, forward right, rear right, rear, rear left, forward left, center (FIG. 5.65b).

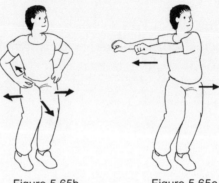

Figure 5.65b   Figure 5.65c

◆ Keep your head, trunk, and pelvis upright and balanced over each other. Reach your arms in the opposite direction from where you are shifting your weight to help maintain your balance (FIG. 5.65c).

◆ Repeat 3-5 times in clockwise and counterclockwise directions.

Multi-Directional Lunging

Why: This exercise is ideal for balance training and benefits overall strength, flexibility, and cardiovascular health to enhance performance in lifting and prevention of injury.

Beginning Position: Stand tall in good posture; identify your neutral spinal alignment. Utilize this position as you perform the four types of lunge patterns.

Movement:

◆ Forward Lunge (FIG 5.66): Focus on lowering your knee toward the floor in a comfortable, controlled range.

◆ Lateral Lunge (FIG 5.67): Focus on keeping your feet pointed forward with your knee following your foot in a comfortable, controlled range.

◆ Rotational Lunge (FIG 5.68): Focus on rotating the lunging foot to point in the direction you are lunging with your knee following your foot in a comfortable, controlled range.

◆ Backward Lunge (FIG 5.69): Focus on lowering the back knee toward the floor in a comfortable, controlled range.

◆ Perform four lunges in each direction for each leg. Each lunge should go progressively further than the previous lunge while remaining in comfortable, controlled ranges.

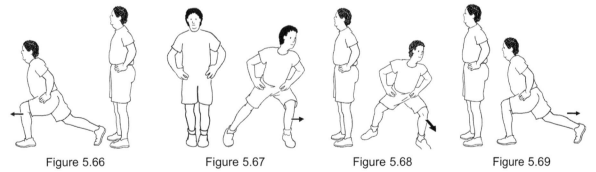

Figure 5.66   Figure 5.67   Figure 5.68   Figure 5.69

▲ *Good Moves:*

▲ Maintain spinal alignment.

▲ Keep your knee following your toe.

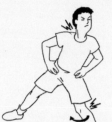

Figure 5.70

▼ *Bad Moves* (FIG. 5.70)*:*

▼ Performing lunges in poor postural alignment, such as slouching or with your chin protruding forward, will stress your neck and back.

▼ Performing lunges too deeply so that the knee moves over the foot or collapses inside of the foot will stress the knee.

Advanced Standing Three Plane Core:

Why: To promote postural awareness and the strength of your trunk (core), legs, and arms so as to improve your squatting, lifting, twisting, and reaching abilities.

> **CAUTION: THESE EXERCISES SHOULD NOT BE PERFORMED IF YOU ARE IN PAIN OR IF THEY PRODUCE PAIN.**

Beginning Position:

◆ Stand with feet shoulder-width apart and turned slightly out.

◆ Keeping your spine aligned, elongate your trunk. Stay in this position as you perform the three movement patterns described below.

◆ Hold onto a ball or other small object at chest height; always return your hands to chest-height position after reaching.

Movements:

◆ Sagittal Core:

• Maintain good alignment as you squat and reach forward toward the floor in a comfortable, controlled range. Focus on gliding your hips backward (Fig. 5.71a). Return to starting position.

• Maintain alignment as you extend and reach overhead and behind you toward the ceiling in a comfortable, controlled range. Focus on gliding your hips forward (FIG. 5.71b). Return to starting position.

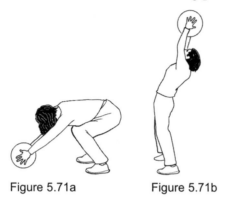

Figure 5.71a   Figure 5.71b

• Repeat this movement 5–20 times.

◆ Frontal Core:

• Maintain good alignment as you reach overhead, bending sideways to the right in a comfortable, controlled range. Focus on your hips gliding to the right (FIG. 5.72a). Return to starting position.

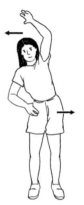

Figure 5.72a

• Maintain good alignment as you reach overhead, bending sideways to the left in a comfortable, controlled range. Focus on your hips gliding to the right (FIG. 5.72b). Return to starting position.

• Repeat this movement 5–20 times.

◆ Transverse Core:

• Maintain good alignment as you twist to the right, reaching your arms out toward the wall behind you

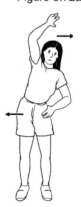

Figure 5.72b

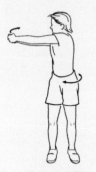

Figure 5.73a

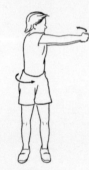

Figure 5.73b

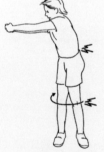

Figure 5.74

in a comfortable, controlled range. Focus on your hips and middle back twisting to help you reach (FIG. 5.73a). Return to starting position.

• Maintain good alignment as you twist to the left, reaching your arms out toward the wall behind you in a comfortable, controlled range. Focus on your hips and middle back twisting to help you reach (FIG. 5.73b). Return to starting position.

• Repeat this movement 5–20 times.

◆ Advanced: To advance these exercises hold heavier objects; start with one pound and slowly increase the load as the movements become easier.

▲ *Good Moves:*

▲ Maintaining good spinal posture is critical to the success of these exercises.

▲ Focus on the motion coming from your hips gliding and your arms reaching.

▼ *Bad Moves:*

▼ Using knee motion rather than gliding your hips puts more stress on your knees and back (FIG. 5.74).

STRENGTHENING USING MACHINES

Weight training of any kind (using machines, free weights, rubberized bands, etc.) involves applying resistance to normal body motions. This can be thought of as a form of mechanical stress. Your body can react in many ways to this stress. Your particular reaction should determine whether this form of exercise is beneficial, a waste of time, or actually harmful for you.

Success Factors

Improving your awareness and control of three basic factors can definitely make your efforts at strengthening much more successful. These factors are your breathing, alignment, and muscle tone.

Breathing:

▲ *Good Moves:*

▲ Maintain relaxed, easy breathing, using inhalation to "buoy you up" and using exhalation to reinforce power.

▲ Take occasional Cleansing Breaths to assist with overall relaxation, release tension build-up in specific areas, and bring your pulse rate down.

▲ Perform slow, deep inhalation through the nose and/or mouth. Pause on the inhale for one second while the "bad air" collects, then exhale through your relaxed, open mouth and release tension and "bad air."

▼ *Bad Moves:* Avoid holding your breath or getting up-tight about breathing at the "right" time. Counting out loud can insure that you are breathing if you tend to hold your breath.

Alignment:

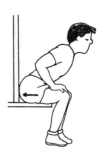
Figure 5.75

▲ *Good Moves:*

▲ Maintain exaggerated good alignment throughout the exercise. For example, when weightlifting while sitting, exaggerate Pelvic Repositioning (FIG. 5.75.)

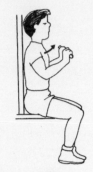

Figure 5.76

so that you are in your most stable, upright position. If the seat feels too deep, use the adjustment for seat depth and move it forward.

▲ Look in the mirror as you lift, pull, or push and make sure you maintain good alignment (FIG. 5.76).

▲ When weightlifting while standing, move your feet shoulder-width apart and maintain a neutral alignment of your spine (tense your lower abdomen) so that your lower back and pelvis remain relatively level and stable as you lift with your arms (FIG. 5. 77).

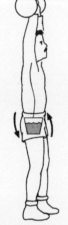

Figure 5.77

▼ *Bad Moves:* Don't let the resistance move you into faulty alignments; this tendency increases when you are tired or attempting to lift too much weight.

Tone:

▲ *Good Moves* (FIG. 5.78):

▲ Attempt to position and move yourself so that you make it look fairly easy and smooth: keep your face/expression relaxed, keep your teeth apart, and use images or thoughts to help you look tranquil and in control.

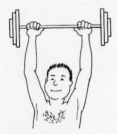

Figure 5.78

▲ Move smoothly and evenly. The rate of motion should be pretty much the same from the beginning to the end of the exercise (approximately three seconds each way). Pause at the completion of the exercise and return to the beginning position with the same control.

▼ *Bad Moves* (FIG. 5.79):

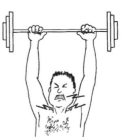

Figure 5.79

▼ Avoid tensing up the front of your neck or raising your shoulders as you use the arms.

▼ Avoid scrunching your face or clenching the teeth together; avoid tensing and pushing up or down through the back or buttocks.

▼ Avoid fast movements, which use momentum and result in problems with alignment, tone, and pain.

How Much/How Often

Do 8–15 repetitions 2–4 times per week. You should be able to do this many repetitions well with moderate effort (not too easy, not too stressful). If in your last few repetitions you cannot manage the complete range of the exercises, or if you begin to "struggle" or drop out of alignment, you are attempting to lift too much weight. If your last few repetitions are just as easy as your first, you are not lifting enough weight. As a starting point or goal, you need not do more than 8–15 repetitions for each exercise, nor is it necessary to do the exercises more than 2–4 times per week. However, if you want to advance your strength and functional potential, the recommendation and goal would be to do 15–25 repetitions. If you are an athlete, the recommendation and goal would be to do 25–35 repetitions.

Example Exercises

The following examples provide general recommendations for quality and safety of movement when using equipment typically found in fitness facilities. Follow the instructions provided with the specific piece of equipment you are using, or consult an exercise professional for instruction in proper use of the equipment.

Quadriceps (front of thigh):

Why: To strengthen the muscles on the front of the thigh, which are important for squatting and lifting, climbing stairs, etc.

▲ *Good Moves* (FIG. 5.80):

▲ Exaggerate Pelvic Repositioning (see pp. 52–53) so that your lower back is relaxed but supported in an arched pattern.

▲ Straighten the knees as far as is comfortable as you remain sitting tall. There should be arm handles underneath your seat to help keep you up tall.

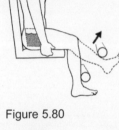

Figure 5.80

▼ *Bad Moves* (FIG. 5.81):

▼ Avoid sitting on your tail so that you begin or end up in a slump.

▼ Avoid straightening your knees fully when you have tight hamstrings; this can result in rounding your back, causing a significant increase in low back compression.

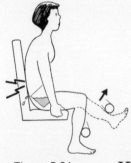

Figure 5.81

Hamstrings (back of thigh and buttocks):

Why: To strengthen the muscles on the back of the thigh, which are important for squatting and lifting, climbing stairs, etc.

Stomach Lying Hamstring Curl

▲ *Good Moves* (FIG. 5.82):

▲ As you bend the knees, keep your groin pressed flat onto the table so that the back stays flat and the buttocks stay down.

▲ Keep the upper back and neck relaxed.

▲ Pull with the arms to assist, and bend the knees as far as you can as long as you maintain a flat low back and buttocks position.

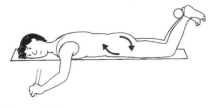

Figure 5.82

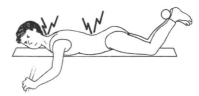

Figure 5.83

▼ *Bad Moves* (FIG. 5.83):

▼ Do not allow the lower back to arch and/or the buttocks to rise up and stick out.

▼ Don't tense up or lift up the head as you bend the knees.

Seated Hamstring Curl

▲ *Good Moves* (FIG. 5.84):

▲ Exaggerate Pelvic Repositioning (see pp. 52–53) so that your lower back is relaxed but supported in an arched pattern.

▲ Bend the knees as far as comfortable as you remain sitting tall. There should be arm handles underneath your seat to help keep you up tall.

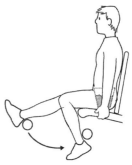

Figure 5.84

▼ *Bad Moves* (FIG. 5.85):

▼ Avoid sitting on your tail so that you begin or end up in a slump.

▼ Avoid any spinal motion at the beginning or end of the movement.

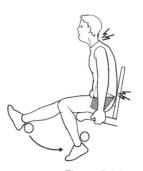

Figure 5.85

Abdominals (stomach muscles):

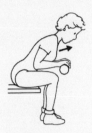

Why: To strengthen abdominal muscles for better posture.

Seated Trunk Curl

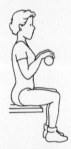

▲ *Good Moves* (FIG. 5.86):

▲ Maintain abdominal muscle tension throughout the movement while keeping a chest-up/head-neutral posture.

▲ Rest your arms up on the machine through the entire motion.

▲ It is not necessary to go through the complete range, especially if this is uncomfortable for your lower back, buttocks, and/or legs.

Figure 5.86

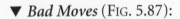

CAUTION: THIS EXERCISE SHOULD NOT BE PERFORMED IF YOU HAVE RECENTLY HURT YOUR BACK.

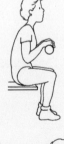

▼ *Bad Moves* (FIG. 5.87):

▼ Do not pull your lower back down into a rounded, compressed pattern.

▼ Do not pull your head forward in front of your chest as you bend down.

▼ Do not pull down using your arms.

▼ Do not look up as you lower your trunk down.

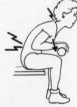

Figure 5.87

Seated Trunk Rotation

▲ *Good Moves* (FIG. 5.88):

▲ Maintain abdominal muscle tension throughout the movement while keeping a chest-up/head-neutral posture.

▲ Maintain the posture as you rotate the trunk, moving from the waist.

▲ Maintain relaxed, easy breathing, using inhalation as you return to the starting position and exhalation as you twist.

▼ *Bad Moves* (FIG. 5.89):

▼ Avoid allowing the lower back to slump into a rounded, compressed pattern.

▼ Avoid allowing your head and neck to fall forward in front of your chest as you twist.

▼ Do not hold your breath as you are twisting.

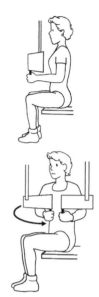

Figure 5.88

Hanging Roman Chair

▲ *Good Moves* (FIG. 5.90):

▲ Maintain abdominal muscle tension throughout the movement while keeping a chest-up/head-neutral posture.

▲ Maintain good posture as you lift your leg toward your chest and lower, making sure the movement is coming from your abdominal area.

▲ Maintain relaxed, easy breathing, using inhalation as you return to the starting position and exhalation to reinforce power as you turn.

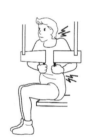

Figure 5.89

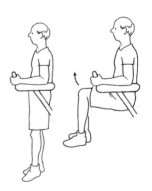

Figure 5.90

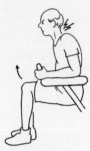

Figure 5.91

▼ *Bad Moves* (FIG. 5.91):

▼ Avoid shrugging the shoulders.

▼ Avoid lifting the leg by arching the back and pushing the head forward.

▼ Avoid turning the knee and foot inward when lifting and lowering your leg.

▼ Avoid moving the legs too quickly or in an uncontrolled manner.

Back Extensors (back muscles):

Why: To strengthen back muscles for better posture.

Back Extension Machine

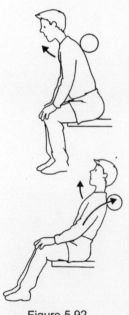

Figure 5.92

▲ *Good Moves* (FIG. 5.92):

▲ Maintain abdominal muscle tension throughout the movement while keeping a chest-up/head-neutral posture.

▲ Lift up and in with your lower abdominals as you push backward with your spine.

▲ Stop at any point in the range where you feel discomfort or pressure in the lower back or legs. Your range of comfortable movement will change with repetition and time—don't try to force it.

CAUTION: THIS EXERCISE SHOULD NOT BE PERFORMED IF YOU HAVE RECENTLY HURT YOUR BACK.

▼ *Bad Moves* (FIG. 5.93):

▼ Avoid starting out or ending up with your lower back slumped, your chest down, and your head forward.

▼ Don't arch the neck backward as you perform this exercise.

Figure 5.93

Back Hyperextension Bench

▲ *Good Moves* (FIG. 5.94):

▲ Maintain abdominal muscle tension throughout the movement while keeping a chest-up/head-neutral posture.

▲ Maintain this posture as you lower your trunk from the hips; make sure the support pad is just under your front pelvic bones.

▲ Maintain relaxed, easy breathing, using inhalation as you lower your trunk and exhalation as you raise your trunk to starting position.

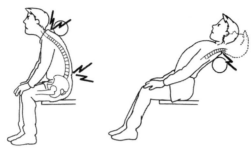

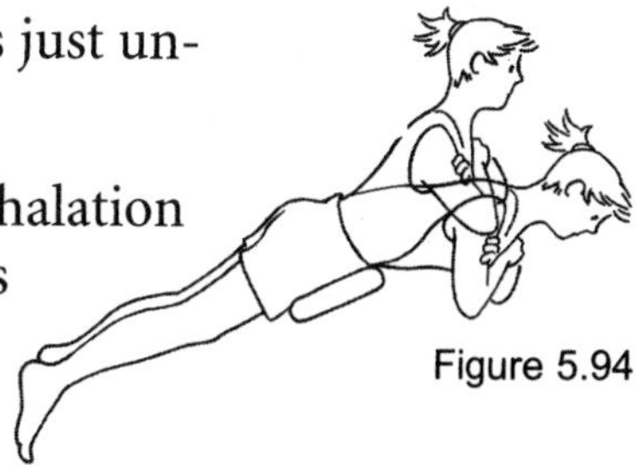

Figure 5.94

▼ *Bad Moves* (FIG. 5.95):

▼ Don't allow the lower back to slump into a rounded, compressed pattern.

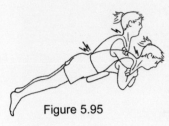

Figure 5.95

▼ Avoid allowing your head and neck to fall forward in front of your chest as you lower and raise your trunk.

▼ Don't allow the support pad to be under your lower abdominal area; this allows for more torque to be distributed to your lower back instead of your hips.

Lats And Shoulder Girdle (upper back muscles):

Why: To strengthen the muscles of the shoulder and upper/lower back, which are used for pulling activities.

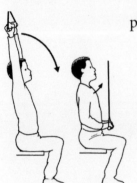

Figure 5.96

▲ *Good Moves* (FIG. 5.96):

▲ Lean your trunk back about 30 degrees and maintain abdominal muscle tension throughout the movement while keeping a chest-up/head-neutral posture.

▲ Initiate the movement by pulling your shoulder blades down and together as your arms move towards your chest.

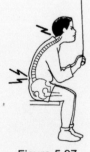

Figure 5.97

▼ *Bad Moves* (FIG. 5.97):

▼ Avoid pulling down with your trunk so that the head is pulled forward and down with the chest.

▼ Avoid arching the head backward as you pull down or sticking your neck out as you pull the bar down.

Deltoids (shoulder muscles):

Why: To strengthen the shoulder muscles used for pushing-up/lifting-up and overhead motion.

▲ *Good Moves* (FIG. 5.98):

▲ Maintain upright sitting alignment throughout the lift and return.

▲ Think of keeping your low back area relaxed, light, and unstressed—this will ensure that your arms are doing the work.

▲ Keep wrists straight during the exercise.

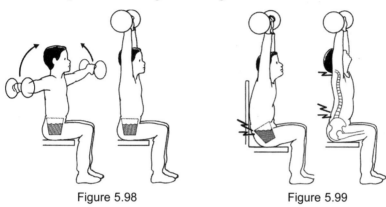

Figure 5.98   Figure 5.99

▼ *Bad Moves* (FIG. 5.99):

▼ Avoid dropping into a slump.

▼ Avoid arching up with the lower back and upper neck to assist with the pushing motion of the arms.

▼ Avoid locking your elbows.

Pectorals (chest muscles):

Why: To strengthen your upper chest muscles, which are used for pulling things in and across the body.

▲ *Good Moves* (FIG. 5.100): Keep your chest up with your head in neutral posture as you pull the arms across your chest.

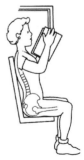

Figure 5.100

▼ *Bad Moves* (FIG. 5.101): Avoid overarching the neck and lower back as you return to the start position.

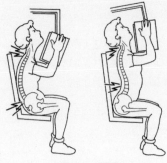

Figure 5.101

Pectorals and Front Deltoids (upper chest and front shoulder muscles):

Why: To strengthen the chest and the front of your shoulders, which are used for pushing things away from your body.

▲ *Good Moves* (FIG. 5.102):

▲ Maintain neutral, relaxed alignment of the head, trunk, and pelvis throughout the motion.

▲ Position your feet on the floor or up on the bench, depending on which position allows you to maintain neutral spinal alignment.

▲ Keep the neck and jaw relaxed as you push up.

▲ Keep wrists straight during this exercise.

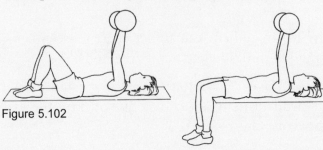

Figure 5.102

▼ *Bad Moves* (FIG. 5.103):

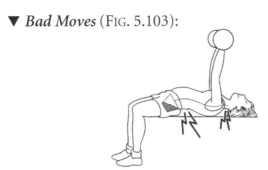

Figure 5.103

▼ Avoid tensing and pushing up with the back and/or neck in an arched or rounded pattern.

▼ Don't press the back of the head or neck onto the bench.

▼ Avoid locking elbows.

Biceps (front upper arm muscles):

Why: To strengthen the muscles in the front of your upper arms, which are important for lifting and pulling.

▲ *Good Moves* (FIG. 5.104 and FIG. 5.105):

▲ Exaggerate maintaining your chest upright.

▲ Keep the head balanced tall and level over the chest.

▲ If standing, keep your feet shoulder-width apart and your pelvic bowl level from front to back.

▲ Keep your upper arms straight by your sides with the elbows supported in front of your torso as you raise and lower your forearm.

▲ Keep your shoulders down and squeeze your shoulder blades together as you lift the weight.

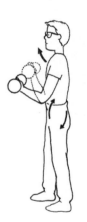

Figure 5.104

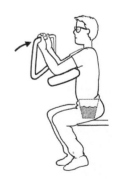

Figure 5.105

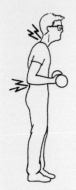

Figure 5.106

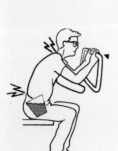

Figure 5.107

▼ *Bad Moves* (FIG. 5.106 and FIG. 5.107):

▼ Avoid dropping the chest and head down in front.

▼ Avoid letting your elbow drift backward behind your shoulders as you raise and lower the weight.

▼ Don't allow the pelvic bowl to tip forward or backward.

▼ Don't shrug your shoulders as you lift the weight.

Triceps (back upper arm muscles):

Why: To strengthen the muscles in the back of your upper arms, which are important for reaching, throwing, or pushing.

▲ *Good Moves* (FIG. 5.108 and FIG. 5.109):

▲ Keep the head balanced tall and level over the chest.

▲ Keep your pelvic bowl level from front to back.

▲ If standing, keep your feet shoulder-width apart, knees slightly bent.

▲ Keep your elbows in.

▲ Keep your wrists straight during this exercise.

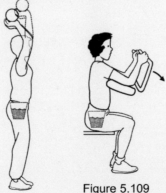

Figure 5.108   Figure 5.109

▼ *Bad Moves* (FIGS. 5.110 and 5.111):

▼ Avoid sticking your chin out or arching your back.

▼ Don't let the elbows drift outward.

▼ Avoid shrugging your shoulders.

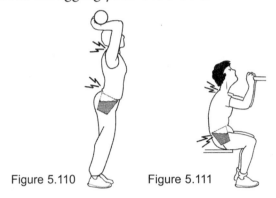

Figure 5.110   Figure 5.111

AEROBIC EXERCISE

What and Why

Aerobic exercise is any activity that is performed at such intensity and rate that oxygen is utilized as the main fuel to produce the energy you need to perform. In order for you to reap the full benefits of aerobic exercise, it must be performed long enough (a total of at least 20–60 minutes, which can be performed in 10-minute intervals), often enough (at least 3–5 times per week), and at the right intensity (within your target heart rate zone). Common examples of possible aerobic exercise forms include fast walking, jogging, biking, swimming, and dancing.

There are a number of reasons why you would benefit from performing a consistent form of aerobic exercise. It can improve the strength and efficiency of your heart and circulatory system, thereby reducing the risk of heart attack, high blood pressure, heart disease, and stroke. It can also improve your overall endurance for activity as well as help you to live healthier and longer. Your body becomes more efficient at using oxygen for energy, and your immune system will be stronger. In addition to these general benefits, aerobic exercise offers four specific benefits to neck and back pain sufferers:

■ It is the healthiest and most effective way to lose weight naturally (it is the only form of exercise that can efficiently metabolize fat cells). In some cases, being overweight can aggravate your pain, so losing weight through aerobic exercise can help.

■ It can assist you with longer-lasting pain relief. It is the only form of exercise that can significantly stimulate production and release of endorphins—the body's potent and natural chemicals that help block the pain circuits.

■ It can also make you less prone to injury and aggravation of your symptoms because it makes your structural system stronger and more flexible.

■ It can improve your self-esteem and help you to decrease feelings of anger, depression, and anxiety, all of which can aggravate your pain symptoms.

All of these potential benefits depend on how you perform the particular aerobic activity that you choose. It is crucial that you choose the type of aerobic activity that is compatible with your system (physically and emotionally) and that you perform it in such a way that you reach the aforementioned goals. This leads to the general question of how best to perform any aerobic exercise.

How Often

The American College of Sports Medicine recommends that aerobic exercise be performed three to five times per week for optimal cardiovascular health. If you don't exercise aerobically at least three times a week consistently, your system won't have a chance to improve its performance. It is important to choose activities that you enjoy and are comfortable doing so that you are more likely to maintain the consistency needed to gain these benefits. Also, sporadically and/or occasionally attempting to perform aerobic exercise is physically stressful and can be risky if done too intensely.

Performing aerobic exercise more than five times a week should be reserved for the dedicated and well-conditioned athlete. Performing aerobic exercise too frequently for your system will typically result in fatigue, less enjoyment, and pain. It may ultimately lead to more serious injury and/or illness as your structural and immune systems get worn down.

How Long

To gain the full benefit of aerobic exercise, the exercise should be maintained for at least 10 minutes at a time, adding up to 20–60 minutes per day. Listen to your system—remember that you're supposed to look and feel good, not worn out. If you are having difficulty increasing the duration of your activity, you are probably working too intensely, too fast. (Check your heart rate to see if this is the problem.) If you attempt to last for longer than 60 minutes of aerobic exercise, especially when first beginning, you may run into the same problems caused by exercising too frequently: your body will "complain" so much that you probably won't attempt to exercise aerobically very often.

How Much

After a 5–10 minute gradual warm-up period, the rate and intensity of your movement should increase, resulting in your pulse rising to your Target Heart Rate (THR). Maintaining your target heart rate for at least 10 minutes is the basis of all aerobic conditioning programs.

Use these simple formulas for determining your THR:

■ 220 minus your age times .55–.65 (beginning exercisers) = THR

■ 220 minus your age times .65–.80 (regular exercisers) = THR

■ 220 minus your age times .80–.90 (advanced exercisers) = THR

The chart below "spells out" the THRs for various age groups:

Age	Beginning Target HR (60%) 220-Age X 60%	Regular Target HR (70%) 220-Age X 70%	Advanced Target HR (85%) 220-Age X 85%
20	120	140	170
25	117	137	166
30	114	133	162
35	111	130	157
40	108	126	153
45	105	123	149
50	102	119	145
55	99	116	140
60	96	112	136
65	93	109	132
70	90	105	128

Checking Your Pulse Rate

Why: To determine whether you are exercising at your THR, you should check your pulse rate (per minute) during, immediately after, and then five to ten minutes after concluding your aerobic exercise. This is especially important when you first start exercising; it will tell you if you are working too hard (over your THR) or not hard enough (under your THR).

During and immediately after aerobic exercise, your pulse rate should be within your THR. Five to ten minutes after aerobic exercise, your pulse rate should be back down at least below 100 beats per minute—if it's not, you may be working too hard! In general, the quicker your pulse rate returns to your normal resting pulse rate, the more physically fit you are.

How: Find your carotid artery by placing your index and middle fingers lightly on your throat above and to the side of your Adam's apple (FIG. 5.112); press into the soft tissue gently until you feel your pulse. Or, find your radial pulse by placing these same fingers over the palm side of your wrist on the thumb side (FIG. 5.113); press gently till you feel your pulse. Now, count the number of pulses that occur over a 10-second period and multiply this number by six to determine your pulse rate per minute. There are also many heart rate monitoring devices available today to help you measure and monitor your heart rate.

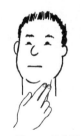

Figure 5.112

If you are working out too hard or too fast, your pulse rate per minute will be over your THR; you will be out of breath, unable to repeat your name and address without gasping for air; you may feel wobbly, dizzy, and probably will look worn out; you may be perspiring excessively; you may look like you're stressed out; etc.

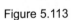

Figure 5.113

If you aren't working out hard or fast enough, your pulse rate per minute will be under your THR; you will be hardly winded, and you'll be able to sing your name and address without gasping for air; you'll feel as if you're not working hard at all, and you'll look like you're taking your time; you may not even be perspiring.

Warm-Up and Cool-Down Periods

It is important to spend 5–10 minutes at the beginning and end of your aerobic workout warming up and cooling down. At the beginning of your workout, you need to warm up slowly and lengthen your tissues to ensure that when you start moving faster, your movement will be safe and efficient. It's like warming up your engine before you ask it to race. Specific recommendations for warm-ups will be given for each specific aerobic activity, but in general it's a good idea to warm up by simply doing the same specific activity at a much slower pace, gradually increasing the rate and range of motion (and, subsequently, your heart rate) until, at about 5–10 minutes, you reach your THR.

The cool-down period is also an important safety factor. It is best to slowly cool your "engine" down after it has been "racing" hard and long. The cool-down may include specific stretching exercises, but typically it will consist of simply slowing down the activity you are performing over a 5–10 minute period so that by the time you stop, your heart rate is down below 100 beats per minute.

Note: During both warm-up and cool-down periods, it will be very helpful to monitor and adjust your breathing pattern. Calming and Cleansing Breaths will help to "feed" your muscles and get rid of the build-up of carbon dioxide. If you are out of breath, you are racing and being inefficient—slow down and take a few Cleansing Breaths to help bring your breathing and "engine" back under control!

Walking

Warm-Up:

Consider this your first and second gear. This "low-gear" rate of walking is most efficient when you first get up after sustained sitting or lying down; it serves to warm up the muscles and lubricate the joints. It's a great form of exercise for short trips, and should be done as a warm-up for aerobic walking.

Attempt to land and move smoothly and easily. Speed up and slow down gradually. Don't "race" your "engine" unless you are adequately warmed up, and avoid abrupt starting and stopping. For a few moments, concentrate on exaggerating upright, balanced alignment as you walk; perform whatever postural adjustments are necessary. Since you've previously been in a sitting position, which tends to bend, shorten, and round you, it's most beneficial to focus on the images that tend to lengthen and decompress you (for example, Head/Chest Floats—see p. 62). Get in the habit of stretching, opening up with your arms, and taking a few Cleansing and Calming Breaths when you first start moving.

Striding and Strengthening:

After 5-10 minutes of warming up, increase your rate of walking until you are striding at a comfortable, brisk pace. Consider this your third to fifth gears. Begin by performing 3–5 steps of each movement described below. At first, maintain a comfortable walking pace. Then, as the exercise becomes easy, progress to performing the movement over more steps and/or at a quicker (brisk) pace, or make the exercise more challenging by carrying weights in your hands. Also, try these exercises, which can be performed anywhere one can walk.

■ Walk with exaggerated forward arm swings.

■ Walk with long strides.

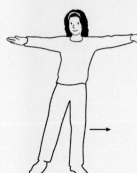

Figure 5.114

■ March, lifting your knees high and extending on your toes.

■ Walk sideways reaching your arms out to your sides going both ways (FIG. 5.114).

■ Walk sideways crossing legs your in front of and behind you while twisting your trunk in opposite ways.

These walking exercises can be used whenever you are able to increase your speed and maintain it. They can improve the strength and flexibility of your entire system. If you are working near your target heart rate for at least 10 minutes, these forms of walking may be the best way for you to improve your aerobic performance. They can be used during everyday commutes and/or specifically as an aerobic exercise program.

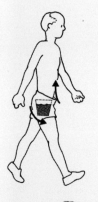

Beware/Be Aware:

At this rate of walking, you may tend to fall into problem alignments or tense your muscles. Instead, make sure you are using the recommendations for healthier walking patterns (see the "Focus on Walking" section of chapter 3). By concentrating on your form, you can increase the number of calories burned and improve your muscle tone.

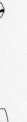

▲ Good Moves While Walking (FIG. 5.115):

▲ **Stay level headed and up tall.** Perform occasional Head/Chest Floats (see p. 62) to help you stay up automatically.

▲ **Keep your pelvis level.** By maintaining a level, stable pelvis as you stride, you naturally strengthen the abdominal and buttocks muscles. Gently lifting up and in with your abdominal muscles for short periods of time (20 seconds to one minute) may be the best and

Figure 5.115

only abdominal exercise you need to do! Maintain a relaxed breathing pattern at the same time.

▲ **Stride forward.** As you bring your leg forward, keep your foot pointed straight ahead or slightly turned outward. Reach with your leg to lengthen your stride. This works the muscles in the front of the leg.

▲ **"Land" and push off correctly.** You should be landing on the outer portion of your heel first, then rolling forward onto the outer side of the foot, and then pushing off with the ball of the foot and the big toe. Concentrate on landing smoothly, without shock. Emphasize pushing off with your calf, back of thigh, and buttocks muscles for increased speed, toning, and calories burned.

▲ **Swing your arms.** Increase the range and rate of your natural arm swing so that it actually assists with propulsion. At moderate speeds, allow your arms to remain fairly straight (elbow slightly bent), swinging like pendulums. At faster speeds, you'll automatically bend your elbows and increase trunk motion to a greater degree to assist with propulsion. By "beefing up" your arm swing in these ways you may burn 5–10 percent more calories. Avoid tensing your shoulders up toward your ears. Avoid twisting or swinging your arms across your body; they should swing forward and back.

Miscellaneous Walking Information:

■ *Walking Shoes:* There are a number of good walking and running shoes available on the market today. It may be helpful for you to go to a store that specializes in running shoes. Make sure you walk around in the shoes for a few minutes and base your decision on comfort, stability of the heel counter, and shock-absorption quality (see pp. 82–84).

■ *Terrain Surfaces:* Surfaces that are smooth with a little "give" to them are the best (for example, running tracks, clay, asphalt, etc.). Keep in mind, though, that these surfaces tend to be angled, so you should alternate direction each time you walk. Harder surfaces (concrete, brick) may aggravate your symptoms due to too much compression, but this problem can be lessened if you wear cushion insoles and shoes with good shock absorption. Walking on soft sand or uneven ground may aggravate your symptoms due to instability and an increased "wobbling" effect, so avoid these surfaces if your pain increases. Progressing to these surfaces, however, can provide a challenge to your system that could help improve your balance.

■ *Hand or Leg Weights:* If you have neck and/or arm symptoms, avoid hand weights; they will tend to pull you down into poor alignment, or tense you up. If you use arm weights, make sure to keep your chest up, your shoulders down, and your neck in good, relaxed alignment. Leg weights will increase your heart rate if you are having difficulty reaching your THR; however, they may tend to make your walking a bit floppy. If you can easily reach your THR without using leg or arm weights, don't bother to use them.

Cross-Country Skiing

This is a great aerobic activity that can be done in the winter splendor of the great outdoors or, if you own a cross-country skiing machine, in the warmth and privacy of your home. The motion is repetitive and fairly simple to master, although it can be a bit tricky at first. It's very similar to the motion of walking; however, the push-off phases for both the legs and the arms are emphasized more than in walking. Cross-country skiing can enhance arm, leg, and trunk strength much more quickly than walking, and perhaps a little more quickly than swimming. There is less risk of injury than during running; and, as in the case of walking, the motion can be particularly beneficial for some low back conditions.

If walking, swimming, or lying flat on your stomach helps decrease your pain, and if you enjoy striding and a sense of winter exhilaration, then cross-country skiing is for you!

If these positions and movements seem to aggravate your symptoms, and/or if you consider walking to be boring and winter a good time to stay in—forget cross-country skiing!

▲ Good Moves (FIG. 5.116):

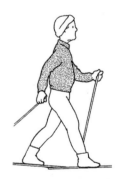

Figure 5.116

    ▲ **Head/neck, chest, and pelvis are in balanced**, upright, and neutral alignment.

    ▲ **Pelvis is kept stable** and is not allowed to tip forward due to your improved awareness and gentle tightening of the lower abdominals and buttocks.

    ▲ **Chest is kept up and open**, allowing for full ventilation and efficient (strong and free) movements of the arms and legs.

    ▲ **Head and neck are balanced** easily on the trunk— they are "going along for the ride," effortlessly following the lead of the chest.

▼ Bad Moves:

▼ Avoid exaggerated alignments and/or tension.

▼ Avoid leading with the head and neck (in front of the chest).

▼ Avoid looking down too much.

▼ Avoid slouching and dropping your chest.

▼ Avoid letting your abdomen and buttocks stick out.

Running

If you've been doing aerobic exercise for some time, you may not be able to get your heart rate up to your THR by walking. Progressing to a slow running program may be an option. Running doesn't always aggravate back and neck pain, but there is a definite increase in the amount of compression to the legs and the spine when you go from walking to running, so be prepared to change aerobic activities if you feel that running is aggravating your symptoms.

All of the information under the "Focus on Walking" section of chapter 3 and the "Walking" and "Cross-Country Skiing" sections of this chapter should be applied here: maintain relaxed tone and balanced alignment of head on trunk and trunk on pelvis, use stable running shoes that offer adequate shock absorption, and run on level, "giving" terrain. Pay special attention to using good form. Running will usually exaggerate any negative postural tendencies that you tend to exhibit while walking; therefore, apply the same methods to decrease these tendencies as covered in previous sections.

▲ Good Moves (FIG. 5.117):

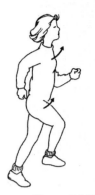

Figure 5.117

▲ **Run level headed and up tall.** Keep your expression relaxed and tranquil—make it look easy! Keep your head level and balanced over your chest. Keep your neck fairly relaxed—imagine that your head is resting on the pedestal of your trunk, being carried forward by your chest, which is leading the motion.

▲ **Keep your chest up, relaxed, and open.** Lift when you inhale, and stay up when you exhale; imagine that your chest is being pulled/lifted up and forward by a cable.

▲ **Shoulders and elbows should be kept down but free,** reaching fairly straight forward and pushing back to boost your momentum. Make them subtly work for you; stabilize and relax your torso in good alignment, keeping it relatively still as you move and work those arms.

▲ **The pelvic bowl should be kept level, stable, and tranquil.** Depending on your postural tendency, you may need to tighten up your lower abdomen and/or buttocks to keep your pelvis from tipping forwards.

▲ **Concentrate on good leg alignment and smooth landing.** Follow the same recommendations given under "Walking."

▲ **Keep the head, chest, and pelvis upright, level, and facing in the same direction.** Imagine that they are boxes being carried forward; do not allow them to twist or jiggle much on each other; feel how your arms and legs are balancing them up tall and level while carrying them forward.

▼ Bad Moves:

▼ Avoid down, tight running: facial tension express-es discomfort/pain, nonenjoyment; head is forward; shoulders are held high and rounded, with elbows stick-ing back behind you; chest is slumped or held down by a tight abdomen; lower back is flat or rounded with your tail under you (FIG. 5.118).

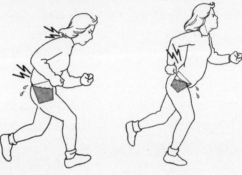

Figure 5.118   Figure 5.119

▼ Avoid uptight running: the same as down, tight running, but with increased arching of the spine, caus-ing the chin, neck, abdomen, and/or buttocks to stick out (FIG. 5.119).

▼ Avoid floppy running: lack of stability and muscle tension causes increased wobbling, twisting, and side-to-side swaying of the head, chest, pelvic bowl, knees, and/or ankles (FIG. 5.120).

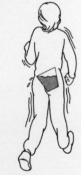

Figure 5.120

Swimming

The great thing about water is that while it supports you and decreases the amount of compression to your joints, it also provides greater resistance to movement so that your muscles work harder the faster you try to move. It's a great way to relax, to strengthen your structure, and to improve your endurance.

▲ Good Moves (FIG. 5.121):

▲ **Think of moving smoothly**, efficiently, and quietly through the water, regardless of the type of stroke you're doing.

▲ **Keep your head and neck in fairly neutral alignment.** For example, when doing the crawl, release the head into the water so that it is facing the bottom of the pool in line with your chest.

▲ **When turning for air, keep your chin in and allow your upper body to turn a bit**, in synch with your head so that the neck is doing a little less turning. If turning your head is still difficult, there are snorkels and other devices to help you maintain neutral alignment of your neck while swimming (FIG. 5.122).

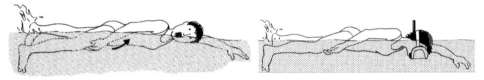

Figure 5.121   Figure 5.122

▲ **Keep your lower back and pelvis in a neutral position** by gently lifting up and in with your lower abdominal muscles.

▲ **If you develop neck or low back pain** from swimming, attempt doing the Knees to Chest, Neck Straightening and Decompression, and Neck Release exercises for relief (see pp. 146–148, 27–31).

▼ Bad Moves (FIG. 5.123):

▼ Avoid holding the head and face up so that the neck is tense and arched up at the top. This postural habit tends to strain the neck as you turn it in order to breathe. Some people do this to keep their hair or eyes from getting wet.

▼ Avoid allowing the lower back to arch excessively so that the abdomen and buttocks stick out. This tends to happen due to the buoyancy of the water, and it will be especially likely to occur if this is your postural tendency outside of the water.

▼ Avoid thrashing, floppy, choppy, unsynchronized movements of the arms and legs. Such movements tend to tip and tilt your head, trunk, and pelvis in various directions, so try to keep the water from splashing.

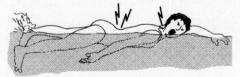

Figure 5.123

Biking

Besides the usual aerobic benefits, this activity is specifically good for loosening up and strengthening the legs. It can be fairly unstressful to the lower back and neck if you are riding in good alignment, on a decent bike, and on fairly smooth surfaces.

▲ Good Moves:

▲ **Stay upright and relaxed by repositioning your pelvis** (see pp. 52–53), taking weight through your arms, keeping your chest up, and maintaining your head in neutral alignment. Use of upright/touring handlebars will help you to stay up in better alignment automatically (FIG. 5.124).

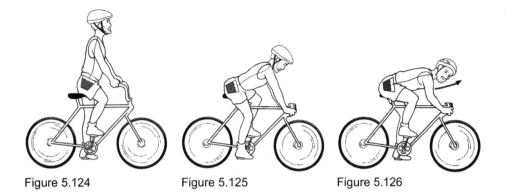

Figure 5.124   Figure 5.125   Figure 5.126

▲ **Proper seat height is important.** When you are pedaling, your down leg should be slightly bent at the hip and knee at the lowest point in the downstroke (FIG. 5.125). If your seat is too high, you will have to tip your pelvis down sideways to reach the pedal at the bottom of your downstroke, causing overarching and twisting of the spine. If your seat is too low, it may encourage slumping, increased compression to the spine, and poor hip and knee form.

▲ **Move and shift positions as needed** for improved comfort. Relax your neck, turn and look to either side, occasionally release your head forward to release/decrease the compression and tension build-up at the base of the skull and upper neck (FIG. 5.126). This is especially important if you are using racing handlebars!

▲ **Keep compression and shock to a minimum.** This may mean turning in your small, firm racing seat for a larger, more supportive model with springs or gel cushioning for greater shock absorption. You might also benefit from various types of seat covers. Some of these are specially designed to reduce pressure and shock. Lambskin covers, etc., are certainly an improvement over a bare seat, but they do not provide as much shock absorption as gel covers. Foam handlebar covers, tape, and padded gloves may help reduce irritation to the arms, neck, or head. If you want an even smoother, shock-free ride, ask your local bike "specialist" about special tires and seat posts with built-in shocks.

Using good form to reduce compression and shock is fairly simple. When the ride gets rough or when you've been sitting too long, shift more weight onto your feet and hands and off your seat; in other words, let the force dissipate through your arms and legs before it reaches your spine. Try "standing" with one leg straight and the other bent up or with both legs fairly straight, leaning a little forward with more weight on your arms. Obviously, do not attempt these movements if you have poor balance to begin with.

If you are having any discomfort, you should add the release and lengthening exercises that you find most helpful (after five minutes of regular cool down). The Neck Straightening and Decompression, Neck Release, Spinal Counter Rotation, and Pressup exercises will probably be most helpful (see pp. 27–29, 29–31, 142–146, 148–149).

▼ Bad Moves (FIG. 5.127):

▼ Avoid hanging your head forward and/or sticking your neck out. These patterns can be avoided by maintaining an upright chest alignment. As soon as the chest is slumped, the head drops forward, so that in order to see the road, you have to tense your neck up, which can quickly lead to soft-tissue and joint irritation. Use of racing handlebars often results in this problem. They're nice if you're into racing, but otherwise, replace your racing handlebars with upright/touring handlebars. If you don't want to replace them, at least make sure that you have your brake handles mounted so you can ride with your hands up on the top of the handlebar.

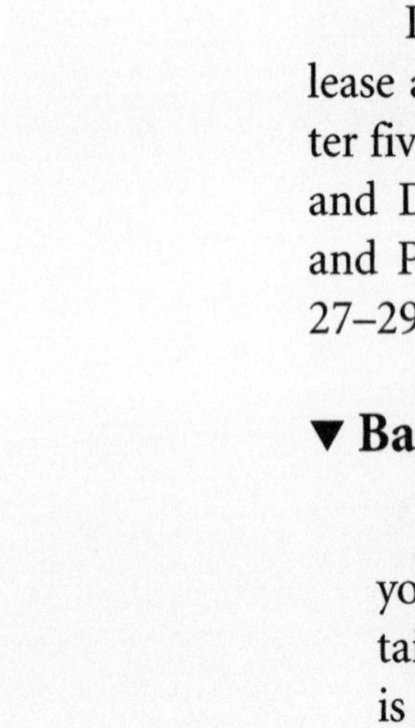

Figure 5.127

▼ Slump biking will add more compression. Sitting with your back rounded and your tail under you can aggravate your condition, especially if you're on a bumpy road. This can occur with any type of handlebar but is especially a common problem when using the racing kind. Check the height of your seat if you tend to exhibit this alignment—it may be too low.

▼ Avoid staying in one position too long without shifting. Whether you are in relatively good or bad alignment, holding or slumping in one position for too long will lead more quickly to strain, fatigue, and discomfort.

Aerobic Dancing

This popular form of aerobic exercise can help strengthen and improve the flexibility of your entire structure. If you are fairly comfortable moving about while standing, and if you like dancing to music, you should try it! If standing and/or raising your arms up seems to aggravate your pain, and/or if you dislike dancing, don't bother trying it.

The most important way to ensure improved strength and comfort of your spine is to maintain good alignment of the head, chest, and pelvis. Bad form is typically a result of moving too fast, lifting the arms and legs too high, hitting down too hard, using bad bending form, and not paying attention to or controlling your general spinal alignment.

Low-Impact Aerobic Dancing

This form of aerobic dancing means that at least one foot is on the ground at all times; hence you do no hopping or jumping, and therefore you subject your body to less shock. You should try this form of aerobic dancing first. If you find that it aggravates your symptoms, don't even try the high-impact classes!

Step aerobics is considered low impact. It involves repetitively stepping up and down off steps of various heights while

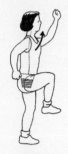

moving your arms out to the sides and overhead. Step aerobics can be excellent if done slowly and with good form. Unfortunately, the emphasis is often placed on speed, which tends to produce bad form (rounding or overarching the lower back, dropping the upper back and neck forward, arching the neck backward).

High-Impact Aerobic Dancing

This form of aerobic dancing allows you to be more "airborne." Because of the wider range of movements involved, some people find it somewhat more fun and invigorating. However, if you think that the increased shock is aggravating your symptoms, switch back to the low-impact classes.

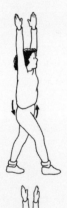

Figure 5.128

▲ Good Moves:

▲ **Exaggerate and maintain your best alignment** while aerobic dancing. Focus on keeping your head, chest, and pelvis balanced, upright, and stable while you move around. Use a mirror to help you monitor and maintain this alignment.

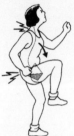

▲ **During forward kicking/raising/marching motions of the legs, focus on keeping your chest up tall**; do not raise your legs up so high or fast that they pull you down into a slouch. Concentrate on smooth, specific motions of the legs, with your head and chest staying up tall and relaxed (FIG. 5.128).

▲ **When moving your arms overhead, keep your head and pelvis level** (see Pelvic Leveling and Head/Chest Float postural adjustments, pp. 71–72, 62). Avoid the tendency to stick or drop your head forward. Avoid sticking out your abdomen and buttocks as the arms go up (FIG. 5.129).

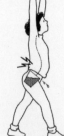

Figure 5.129

▲ **Keep your legs in good alignment.** Keep your knee joints balanced over the middle of your feet. Whether you are marching, lunging, or squatting, your knee should be facing in the same direction as your foot and should be positioned directly over it. Never let your knee move forward past your foot!

▲ **Attempt to land lightly and smoothly.** Whether you are hitting down on the balls of your feet or more toward the heel, you can take some of the shock out by simply trying to land more quietly. Check out some of the newer models of shoes designed specifically for aerobics—they should have stable heel counters and good shock absorption quality.

▲ **Do your aerobic dancing on stable, level surfaces that have some "give" to them,** such as wood, rubberized surfaces, or specially padded "aerobic" floors. Concrete and shag carpeting are not good surfaces for aerobic dancing.

▼ Bad Moves:

▼ Avoid bending forward from a standing position with your legs straight. These movements are potentially harmful, and they serve no positive health benefit! So if the rest of the class is doing floor or toe touches, substitute partial squatting with your feet wide apart during these class periods. This will improve your leg strength and flexibility while improving the stability of your spine.

▼ Avoid overworking. It is common for many people to be dancing far above their THR. This is not aerobics; rather, it is a negative physical stress that the body will not appreciate! One of the problems of following an instructor or a class is that you may try to keep up with their rate and duration of movement rather than listening to your own system. You must monitor your own system and slow down your movements when needed to ensure that you are around your own THR.

▼ Beware of the overzealous instructor or self-induced peer pressure. Yes, instructors and peers can help you with motivation, but don't be overconcerned with moving faster, kicking higher, or staying synchronized with the class. Listen and watch your system in the mirror—do what you need to do to improve your immediate posture and tone (muscular and emotional). Sometimes this means doing different exercises than the class—ones that can keep you around your THR but do not aggravate your pain.

▼ Beware of marathon aerobic sessions unless your system can handle them positively. Many aerobics classes last an hour. This usually includes a warm-up and cool down. This is fine if you're ready for about 40 minutes of aerobic activity, but not if you're just starting out! In the beginning, don't expect your system to be capable of more than 10 minutes of exercise (at your THR).

Alternative Exercise Methods

There are many different ways to exercise in addition to the ones mentioned here. Machines such as treadmills, stair climbers, elliptical trainers, rowers, and cross-country ski machines offer additional varieties of aerobic exercise. Other popular exercise methods include pilates, yoga, tai chi, cardio-boxing, "spinning," aquatic exercise classes, dance classes (ballroom, swing, salsa, etc.), and others. There are no absolute rules about which of these methods are "good" or "bad" for people with back pain. Any activity that helps you lengthen or strengthen your muscles or improve your overall fitness can be beneficial as long as you keep in mind the basic principles discussed throughout this book:

■ You should be able to maintain correct posture (neutral alignment of your spine) throughout the activity.

■ You should be able to maintain a steady breathing pattern throughout the activity.

■ You should be generally comfortable throughout the activity and not experience an increase in your back or neck pain from doing it.

You are more likely to stick with an activity that you enjoy, so if you find one that you like and you can maintain these principles while doing it, go for it!

CONCLUSION

The major goal of this book has been to provide you with methods of self-treatment—good moves related to posture, body mechanics, breathing, imagery, and exercise, as well as other strategies for pain control. If at this point you still have questions, if you feel the need for further direction, or if you suspect you need a "hands-on" approach, it is recommended that you consult with a physical therapist experienced in the care of people with neck or back pain. Even if you do not undertake a complete course of physical therapy, a consultation visit may assist you in developing a good self-care program.

There are many ways to locate a physical therapist. You might start by asking your friends, family, coworkers, and physician to recommend physical therapists with whom they have had positive working experiences. You can also call your state or national branch of the American Physical Therapy Association (APTA). They can provide you with names of local therapists. Another approach is to find out if there is a physical-therapy school at your local university. If so, its office can often provide information regarding where to contact an experienced local therapist. Your local hospital probably has a physical therapy department, and there probably are private practice physical therapy groups in your area. If you are not sure about your insurance coverage for physical therapy, you should be able to get this information by calling the claims department of your insurance company.

After performing a detailed evaluation, your physical therapist should be able to provide you with any of the following: specific postural and movement recommendations; pain relief positions, movements, and "blankets" (electrotherapy, traction, corsets, heat, cold, etc.); exercises to improve your flexibility, strength, and endurance; and/or hands-on soft-tissue and joint mobilization techniques to help balance your structural and electrical systems.

In closing, it is up to you to take control of your body and its pain. This book offers you the raw material to begin performing good moves and decrease the incidence of bad moves in your daily life. Hold onto those recommendations that seem to help alleviate your pain. Give your body time to learn these methods and time to heal.

GLOSSARY

---

aerobic—refers to activities in which oxygen is used as the main fuel to produce the energy you need to perform. Aerobic activities are specifically helpful in metabolizing fat cells and improving your body's production and release of beta endorphins (chemical pain relief). Aerobic exercise is generally recommended at least three times a week, with at least 10–60 minutes during which your heart rate stays around your Target Heart Rate. Classic examples include walking, running, and biking, as long as the proper intensity and duration are maintained.

anaerobic—refers to activities performed at such a high intensity or rate that oxygen cannot provide the needed fuel fast enough; classic examples include heavy weightlifting or running the hundred-yard dash. Anaerobic activities can help strengthen you but may aggravate your pain if they are too intense.

base of support—while standing, your base of support would include the area directly under and between your feet. If your feet tend to be placed close together, you have a narrower base of support; this may result in more energy expenditure, muscle tension, and/or strain forces. If your feet tend to be placed further apart (side-to-side or front to back), you have a wider base of support; this may result in less energy expenditure, muscle tension, and strain forces. When standing in one area for a while, or whenever bending, you'll want to increase your base of support by moving your feet apart.

body "blocks"—refers to imagining the body as a series of boxes or blocks stacked on top of each other. Each large segment represents a block: for example, each foot is a block, each thigh is a block, the pelvis is a block, the trunk is a large block that includes the chest and back, etc. Visualizing these blocks assists with improving your alignment, especially while standing and walking.

cardiovascular—refers to the system that includes your heart, arteries, and veins (circulatory system). The health of this system is greatly improved by aerobic activity.

cervical region—refers to the neck area from the base of the skull to the shoulder girdles in back, around the sides of the neck to the throat, and around the front of the neck and down to the collarbones.

comfort circuits—electrical circuits that carry comfort messages in the body. These circuits can be set off by positive thoughts and breathing patterns, good posture and body mechanics, use of relief "blankets," and balanced activity and rest cycles.

compression—describes the pressure of gravity on the body's structural system. The forces of gravity are increased due to poor posture and/or muscle tension, both of which can be aggravated by cold, pain, anger, fear, or depression. Over time, high levels of compression can cause increased wear and tear on the structural system, making it more vulnerable to injury and pain.

contraction—muscle activity creates tension known as a contraction. At rest, and in most stationary positions, there should be only relaxed, low-level contractions occurring to keep the body balanced and supported.

decompression—describes the reduction of pressure on the body's structural system. Compression is reduced by good posture and relaxed muscles. When pain has increased due to your being up too long and doing too much, use of recumbent relief positions (see chapter 3) assists with decompression of the spine and pain relief.

degenerative—refers to structural changes that have occurred because of aging, trauma, and/or disease; in reference to the spine, this might mean narrowing between the vertebrae.

electrical system—a simple way of looking at your nervous system. The electrical system includes your brain, spinal cord, and all the nerves in your body, including the comfort circuits and the pain circuits. Functions of the electrical system include breathing, thinking, and feeling.

endorphins—chemicals produced naturally within the body that assist in blocking the pain circuits. Production and release of endorphins can be facilitated by positive imagery and aerobic activity; it can be inhibited by the long-term use of narcotic pain medications.

ergonomic design—used to describe user-friendly products, such as adjustable office chairs, whose design is based on the structure of the human body as it performs specific functions. Unfortunately, the term "ergonomic design" has become a popular marketing term and is now about as meaningful as "luxury condo."

exaggerated good alignment—as you perform the postural adjustment exercises, your body will move from poor alignment to this alignment. Exaggerated good alignment represents almost an overcorrection of your postural alignment that you consciously hold and look at for short periods of time (10–30 seconds); this overcorrection will help to change your postural "computer" so that it learns that this improved alignment is you. This way, when you relax and let go of holding yourself in the exaggerated good alignment, your body will return to a more neutral improved alignment; that is, it will not return totally to your poor alignment for a while. Over time, by repeating the postural adjustment exercises that move you into exaggerated good alignment numerous times on a daily basis, you will change your posture toward this improved alignment.

extensor muscles—back muscles alongside and overlying the spine, which run from the tailbone up to the base of the neck. When strong, these muscles help to support us up into tall, erect postures. They run on the opposite side of the body from the abdominals, but they work along with the abdominals as "guide wires" to help keep the spine strong and mobile. When weak and stretched out, they tend to allow slumping while sitting, standing, or bending. It they are tight in the low back or upper neck region, increased lordosis and backward arching may occur.

isometrics—refers to muscle contractions where no movement takes place. Tension is developed in the muscle without the muscle being shortened or lengthened.

let-go tests while sitting and standing—these tests involve producing your exaggerated poor alignment by essentially letting go and allowing yourself to view your worst alignment. These tests are not meant to be repeated as an exercise; use them only in the beginning, till you are aware of your exaggerated poor alignment; after that, perform your postural adjustment exercise by simply sitting or standing in your comfortable alignment and then proceeding directly to your exaggerated good alignment.

lordosis (cervical and lumbar)—a natural backward arching of the spine that occurs in these two areas (see Fig. 1.13). A certain degree of curvature is necessary for upright positioning and dissipation of shock; however, pain can result if the lordosis becomes exaggerated, flattened, or actually reversed.

lumbar region—low back area made up of the five lumbar vertebrae, discs, and related soft tissues; area of the back below the thoracic curve and above the pelvis.

lumbar supports—crescent-shaped pillows that assist in supporting the pelvis and lumbar spine up in a straighter position when sitting back against a backrest.

muscle tension—describes muscle activity that results in pain from compression or inflammation. This can be negatively influenced by poor posture, fatigue, and/or negative thoughts and emotions.

muscle tone—describes normal muscle activity in a balanced structural and electrical system during activity and rest.

neutral alignment of the spine—refers to the optimal balance of the head, spinal curves, and pelvis from front to back and side to side. You achieve neutral position by getting into exaggerated good alignment, then gradually relaxing; the resulting improved alignment is your neutral position for the time being. It can gradually improve over time.

overarched lower back—when you look at yourself from the side, your lower back would be considered "overarched" if it is arched so far backward that it causes the lower abdomen and the buttocks to stick out.

overarched neck—when you look at yourself from the side, your neck would be considered "overarched" if it appears to be arched so far backward that it causes your chin to stick up and out, your throat to stretch up and forward, and the top of your head to tip backward. This posture causes significant strain to the neck.

pain circuits—electrical circuits that carry pain messages in the body. These circuits can be set off by negative thoughts and breathing patterns, poor posture and body mechanics, and too much or too little activity.

pelvic tilt—a movement of the lower spine and pelvis in a backward direction causing a flattening of the lumbar curve. The movement is achieved by pulling the abdominal muscles in toward the spine.

range—refers to the amount of movement. In general you should avoid moving into ranges of movement that are uncomfortable or painful; on the other hand, you should attempt to move as far as you can into the ranges illustrated as long as you are comfortable and moving with good alignment.

referred pain—pain felt in a location separate from the source of the pain; for example, pain felt in the thigh, leg, and/or foot due to a back problem, or pain felt in the shoulder, arm, and/or hand due to a neck problem.

rounded-out lower back—when you look at yourself from the side, your lower back would be considered "rounded out" if it appears flat to rounded forward, causing the chest to slump forward. This posture causes a significant increase in compression to the lower back and strain to the neck.

soft tissue—includes tissues of the musculoskeletal (structural) system other than bone—that is, muscles, tendons, ligaments, fascia, discs, cartilage, etc. These tissues are most typically involved in the injury site of musculoskeletal-based pain.

strain forces—compression or stretching that results in moving the body too far or in such a way that some part of it is placed under too much stress.

structural balance—refers to good, symmetrical posture that has a balance of alignment, strength, flexibility, and endurance. If balanced from front to back and side to side, the structure requires minimal use of muscle energy to maintain itself.

structural imbalance—refers to poor, asymmetrical posture that exhibits imbalances of alignment, strength, flexibility, and endurance. The imbalanced structure requires increased muscle tension to maintain itself and suffers greater wear and tear.

structural system—a simple way of looking at your musculoskeletal system. Your structural system includes your skeleton, muscles, tendons, ligaments, etc. Functions controlled by the structural system include posture and body movement during activity, rest, and exercise.

thoracic curve—a slight, long rounding of the spine that occurs below the cervical region and above the lumbar region (see Fig. 1.13). Significant changes in the size or shape of the thoracic curve can result in pain to the neck and lower back.

ventilation—refers to the use of conscious breathing and imagery to assist with relaxation of muscular and nervous tension.

vertebrae—the individual building blocks of the spine (seven cervical, twelve thoracic, five lumbar) that, along with related soft tissues, provide stability, movement, and housing for the spinal cord.

Index of Good Moves

This index provides the page number(s) on which the most complete description is given for the following positions, exercises, postural adjustments, postural supports, let-go tests, relief "blankets," and relief breathing patterns. Please see the table of contents at the front of the book for any movements or sets of movements not listed here.

NOTES

List below the positions or functions that you suspect most often aggravate your pain (see chapters 3, 4, and 5 for ideas).

NOTES

Notes

List below the page numbers of the relief positions (see chapter 2) and postural recommendations (chapters 3 and 4) that are most closely related to your problem positions, movements, or functions.

NOTES

NOTES

Make a list of the exercises that, according to their descriptions in chapter 5 as well as earlier recommendations, sound as if they may have a beneficial effect on you.

NOTES

NOTES

NOTES

NOTES

NOTES